C000117139

MORE EARLY PRAISE FOR
THE ANTI-VIRAL GUT

"Dr. Robynne Chutkan's deep expertise and ability to translate the most cutting-edge science come together in her important new book. It's the actionable plan we all need not just to survive, but to thrive and flourish during this new pandemic era."

—Frank Lipman, MD, coauthor of the *New York Times* bestselling *The New Health Rules*

"Robynne Chutkan is the fairy godmother of the microbiome. She shows us that our gut is *tough* when we treat it right—it can protect us and keep us happy and thriving. Good health begins from within! This book shows us how to keep our defenses strong."

—Jane Esselstyn and Ann Crile Esselstyn, coauthors of *The Prevent and Reverse Heart Disease Cookbook* and *Be a Plant-Based Woman Warrior*

"*The Anti-Viral Gut* provides simple ways to strengthen our natural defenses by catering to the needs of our microbial ecosystem through diet, mind-directed strategies, and healthy lifestyle choices. On the heels of one of the worst viral pandemics in history—and with others on the horizon—this book will provide you with the tools and strategies you need to protect yourself."

—Emeran Mayer, MD, author of *The Gut-Immune Connection*

The
Anti-Viral
Gut

Tackling Pathogens
from the Inside Out

ROBYNNE CHUTKAN, MD

Avery
an imprint of Penguin Random House
New York

AVERY

an imprint of Penguin Random House LLC
penguinrandomhouse.com

Most Avery books are available at special quantity discounts for bulk purchase
for sales promotions, premiums, fund-raising, and educational needs. Special
books or book excerpts also can be created to fit specific needs. For details, write
SpecialMarkets@penguinrandomhouse.com.

Library of Congress Cataloging-in-Publication Data

Names: Chutkan, Robynne, author.
Title: The anti-viral gut: tackling pathogens from the inside out / Robynne Chutkan.
Description: New York: Avery, an imprint of Penguin Random House, [2022] |
Includes index.
Identifiers: LCCN 2022017250 (print) | LCCN 2022017251 (ebook) |
ISBN 9780593420836 (hardcover) | ISBN 9780593420843 (epub)
Subjects: LCSH: Gastrointestinal system—Microbiology. |
Gastrointestinal system—Immunology. | Viruses—Inactivation. |
Medical virology.
Classification: LCC QR171.G29 C48 2022 (print) | LCC QR171.G29 (ebook) |
DDC 612.3/2—dc23/eng/20220808
LC record available at https://lccn.loc.gov/2022017250
LC ebook record available at https://lccn.loc.gov/2022017251

Printed in the United States of America

1st Printing

Book design by Silverglass Studio

*Let us come together to learn from the past,
understand the present, and prepare for the future.*

Contents

PART 3 STRENGTHENING FROM WITHIN—
THE ANTI-VIRAL GUT PLAN

Introduction

It is more important to know what sort of person has a disease than to know what sort of disease a person has.

—**Hippocrates**

On January 20, 2020, the British-registered *Diamond Princess* departed Yokohama, Japan. Five days after leaving port, an eighty-year-old man on board disembarked to seek medical attention for a fever and cough. One week later, Hong Kong officials announced that the passenger, Mr. A, had pneumonia as a result of infection with SARS-CoV-2, the virus that causes COVID. The *Diamond Princess* outbreak represents the kind of experiment we can't do in real life: put a variety of people together in close quarters, expose them to a novel and highly contagious virus, and see what happens next. Ultimately, one in five people on board would become infected, with a fatality rate of about 2 percent. Those numbers, particularly the small but significant percent who died, and the larger unknown number who survived but continued to have symptoms lead us to one of the most important questions of this and future pandemics: Why them?

Why do some people suffer from severe and even fatal forms of viral illnesses like COVID, while others experience only mild symptoms or none at all? Why, despite repeated exposure, do some people never get infected? What determines who makes a complete recovery and who ends up plagued with post-viral "long-haul" symptoms? Is all of this just random luck, or are there important clues that could have predicted who would walk off the *Diamond Princess* and who would leave horizontally?

Those outcomes might seem random, but I assure you, they rarely are. Being on the winning team when battling viruses isn't because of good luck, or coincidence, or variations in viral virulence. It's due to differences in us, the hosts, and our defenses, and those differences are what determine your outcome. Put another way: it's less about the potency of the pathogen and more about the health of the host.

The idea that host health matters as much as or even more than the virulence of the pathogen is validated every day by people who get up close and personal with viruses and never get sick. Even dangerous viruses like Ebola are able to successfully attack only about one in every three adults they come into contact with, and just a tiny percentage of children. In 0.5 percent of people, poliovirus crosses their gut lining, infects their nervous system, and causes crippling paralysis, while in the vast majority who are infected, it causes no symptoms at all. Even today with our arsenal of antiretroviral drugs, HIV can be a death sentence for some, while others live with the virus for years and never develop AIDS. Even more incredibly, about one in ten people are completely immune to HIV and will never become infected, even with repeated exposure.

It may seem like an outlandish idea that you, not the virus, are in the driver's seat, but it's really just common sense when you think about it. Healthy people avoid or recover from life-threatening conditions all the time, while the less hardy and infirm succumb to minor ones. That's true for cancer, heart attacks, viral infections, and virtually every other illness. Increased susceptibility and poor outcomes are in fact almost always predictable and preventable, or at the very least, forecastable and reducible. Simple risk factors assessed in an annual physical, such as blood pressure, cholesterol levels, blood sugar, weight, and smoking status, are extraordinarily accurate in predicting risk for coronary artery disease and heart attacks. And counseling and strategizing about that risk and how to reduce it are much more effective than any drug or medical intervention. It boils down to addressing vulnerabilities and optimizing your body's defensive capabilities. Unfortunately, we're so alienated from our own innate host defenses that we've become dependent on pharmaceuticals as the only solution. Medications are critically important for those who need them, but for the majority of us, our body's own ability to resist, heal, and recover from viruses is vastly superior.

This pandemic has opened our eyes wide to the importance of knowing how to fortify ourselves. COVID-19 has been the deadliest viral outbreak the world has seen in more than a century, but events like it aren't as statistically rare as you may think. A 2021 study from Duke University used records from past outbreaks to estimate the likelihood of them happening again and found the probability of a pandemic like COVID-19 recurring is about 2 percent in any year. That means someone born in 2000 would have about a 40 percent chance of experiencing one by now. The data also shows that the risk of these extreme outbreaks is growing rapidly. Based on the rate at which pathogens like SARS-CoV-2 have erupted in human populations in the past fifty years, the study estimates that novel disease outbreaks will likely grow threefold in the next few decades. At least thirty previously unknown viruses for which no cures are available have been identified in the last half century, including HIV, Ebola, hepatitis C, and now SARS-CoV-2. The reasons for these outbreaks are varied and complex, but most scientists agree that modifications to our food system, climate change, population growth, and more frequent contact between humans and disease-harboring animals are at least partly to blame. Now more than ever, it's critically important for us to understand the direct link between gut health and vulnerability to viruses.

As viruses become more common, exposure to them is inevitable, but illness is not. It all depends on your terrain—your internal ecosystem, or "soil," that nourishes everything in your body, including your immune system—and on having a clear and accurate understanding of what "healthy" really means. The composition and overall health of that soil are more strongly predictive of outcome when you encounter a virus than any other characteristic, including age or the presence of comorbidities like heart disease or obesity. That soil is your microbiome—the trillions of bacteria and other microorganisms that live in your gut and serve as copilots for pretty much every one of your important bodily functions: digestion, synthesis of hormones and vitamins, metabolism of drugs, removal of toxins, communication with your central nervous system, gene activation, and most important, training your immune system to mount just the right balanced response that can effectively clear a virus while avoiding an exaggerated reaction that can damage tissues.

The majority of your immune system is also located in your gut, so it's no surprise that the microbes on one side of your gut lining and the complex immune responses happening on the other are interdependent. If you want to have an immune system that can protect you, even in the face of persistent viral exposure, you must pay attention to what's going on in your gut, because without a healthy and balanced microbiome, your immune system can't do its job properly.

Having an anti-viral gut isn't super complicated. It doesn't involve restricting multiple food groups or taking a bunch of different supplements. It's mostly about being aware and staying clear of the things that interfere with your virus-slaying machinery. That means discontinuing practices that are damaging to your gut microbes; preventing "leaks" in your gut lining that can allow viruses to penetrate and gain access to your internal organs; maintaining adequate amounts of stomach acid that can inactivate viral proteins; making sure the mucus that's produced in your gut is healthy enough to trap and expel viral invaders; understanding the role of fever in halting viral replication; avoiding unnecessary antimicrobials that wipe out your bacterial foot soldiers; not sabotaging your immune system with too much stress and not enough sleep; and, of course, feeding your army of microbes the right stuff so they can do their job of keeping you safe from viruses. It all starts and ends with your gut. In the third part of the book I'll take you through the specific steps to ensure yours is optimized and ready to protect you.

It's disheartening to realize that a hundred years after the last global pandemic, there's so little focus on what individuals can do to increase their resilience to infection, despite the mountain of scientific evidence validating these simple methods for improving host defenses. Our individual and collective health relies on taking action because the reality is that most of us are eventually going to encounter SARS-CoV-2—and other viruses. Public health measures like vaccines and social distancing remain critically important, but strengthening your immune system by optimizing your gut microbiome is arguably *the* most effective strategy for safeguarding yourself and provides an additional layer of protection that ensures that if you are infected, you have the very best outcome.

There's a direct link between the medications you take, your diet and lifestyle, your microbiome, and your immune system, and understanding those relationships is an essential part of building a strong shield against viruses. The good news is that unlike your genes, which are more static, your microbiome is constantly changing, responding dramatically to shifts in your diet within as little as thirty hours of the food hitting your gut. And dietary changes don't just alter the composition of your gut bacteria—they also affect which of your disease-fighting

genes get turned on or off by those bacteria, influencing your susceptibility to infection via genetic mechanisms. Simple changes in environment can have a profound anti-viral effect, too: recuperating outside in
the fresh air during the Spanish flu epidemic of 1918 reduced death
rates from 40 percent to 13 percent, as a direct result of the germicidal
properties of what we now refer to as the open-air factor.

I love animals, but I'm not one of those crazy people who thinks
she can go into the lion's den at the zoo, make friends with the lion,
and walk out unharmed. I'm not a magical thinker; I'm a doctor who
believes in science. And science has shown us what our vulnerabilities
are when it comes to infections like COVID. Despite the virus being
novel, that science is not new. It's the science of gut health, immunity,
and the microbiome. I've used that science in my medical practice to
improve the lives of thousands of patients who suffer from immune-
based gut disorders, and I know how to make it work for you. You can
improve your resistance to viruses, even if you're elderly, sickly, or
have multiple chronic medical problems. You may not be able to make
yourself completely invincible, but by strengthening your gut-based
defenses, you can dramatically improve your chances of surviving
this—and the next—pandemic intact and in even better health. Hippocrates famously said that all disease begins in the gut. Whether
you're trying to prevent infection, recovering from a recent viral illness, or dealing with chronic post-viral symptoms, some of the most
important solutions are to be found there, too.

To view the scientific references cited in this chapter, please visit
drrobynnechutkan.com/anti-viral-gut-references.

HOW IT WORKS

PART 1

The Gut-Immune Connection

By creating an artificial environment, we're not stimulating our immune system enough. Germs are immune stimulants. They challenge you to be prepared.

—Deepak Chopra

Our gut microbes have been evolving with us for a long time—we can trace their origins to a common ancestor more than fifteen million years ago, but our formal understanding of these tiny creatures dates to the 1600s, when the Dutch scientist Antoni van Leeuwenhoek first looked at his own dental plaque under the microscope and saw "little living animalcules." A few centuries later, in the 1800s, the French chemist Louis Pasteur proposed his "germ theory" that certain diseases are caused by the invasion of the body by microorganisms and avoiding contact with them is the way to stay healthy. (It's hard to believe that prior to these groundbreaking findings, people thought foul odors or "evil spirits" were the cause of illness.)

This concept of avoiding germs like the plague has become foundational to modern Western medicine and is the driving force behind our efforts to find new and more effective ways to assault dangerous bugs, like the development of antibiotics and vaccines—discoveries that save countless lives every day. We've formulated medications like monoclonal antibodies that can help us combat viruses and illness if our bodies aren't strong enough to fight them naturally and instituted widespread precautions to keep ourselves protected from pathogens. And simple yet important innovations in sanitation and hygiene, like Florence Nightingale's introduction of handwashing into British army hospitals during the Crimean War, combined with social distancing and quarantining, have also become effective ways of limiting infectious outbreaks.

But as we've decreased the amount of germs on our bodies and in our environment, something else has increased at an alarming rate— and that's our susceptibility to viruses. The increased risk of viral infection includes completely new ones like human immunodeficiency virus (HIV), as well as reemerging oldies like measles, and more transmissible and deadlier versions of some we were already familiar with, like coronavirus. And with COVID-19, we have seen how a global pandemic can impact our daily existence. This paradox of increased infection as we get rid of germs isn't really a paradox at all— it's confirmation of the critical role our microbes play in protecting us from viruses.

THE HIDDEN WORLD INSIDE YOU

Since the days of Leeuwenhoek and Pasteur, we've also made another incredibly important discovery: not all germs are bad! In fact, the trillions of microbes that call our body home are primarily helping rather than hindering us, with a specific purpose that's very much aligned with our own survival. Without these microscopic critters, your immune system wouldn't be able to protect you from infections or cancer; your heart, lungs, and liver wouldn't function properly; and you wouldn't be able to digest food, assimilate nutrients, or synthesize essential vitamins and growth factors that your body can't make on its own. Even your mental health would take a major hit because of the lack of neurotransmitters that microbes produce and the close and necessary interaction between bacteria in your gut and your brain health and development. Why is understanding the relationship we have with our microbes so important? Because these organisms are in fact intimately involved in every aspect of our health—and they're especially critical for protecting us from viruses. Viruses can't survive on their own. They rely on their host's cellular machinery to allow them to live, reproduce, and go on to infect other hosts—a process known as replication. How easily they're able to hijack that machinery is what determines your outcome when infected with a virus, and that is in turn dependent on the trillions of microbes that inhabit your body. To understand how it all works, let's take a closer look at this hidden world inside you.

MULTIPLE MICROBIAL PARTS

The microbiome refers to all the organisms that live in or on your body—from your scalp to your toenails and everywhere in between, but mostly in your gut. This diverse universe includes bacteria, viruses, fungi, protozoa, helminths (worms, for those of us who have them), as well as all their genes. A staggering hundred trillion microbes that include thousands of different species inhabit your body— with more than a billion bacteria in just one drop of fluid in your colon alone. We are single individuals, but we're composed of multiple living, breathing, moving microbial parts.

To appreciate the role and function of your microbes, you can think of your body as a factory. Organs like your lungs, heart, and liver represent the machinery that keeps production moving: extracting oxygen, pumping blood, removing toxins, synthesizing hormones, and performing all of the other complicated tasks that keep us alive. Some of these tasks are automated, but most of the assembly lines require constant monitoring, maintenance, and adjustment. We house the machinery, but who operates it? How does a complex process like, for example, digestion, actually happen? How does the food get broken down into its basic constituents and carried across the gut lining into the bloodstream, where it can be transported to cells that utilize it as an energy source? Who helps produce the substances your body requires but can't make on its own, like the B complex vitamins B_{12}, thiamine, and riboflavin, and vitamin K? How does your body distinguish between serious infection with a dangerous virus and colonization with a harmless one? How does your immune system know when to rally the troops to defend you, and when to ignore benign intruders that don't pose a threat? Your microbes are the ones carrying out all of these tasks—and more! They even turn your genes on and off, activating those you need and dismantling those you don't.

Like David Vetter, the famous "boy in the bubble" who had a disease that weakened his immune system, you'd have to live in a sterile and isolated environment with no contact with the outside world in order to survive without your multitude of microbes, and even that wouldn't be enough to keep you alive because of all the other necessary functions your microbes perform. Since you're their host and they rely on you for their survival, most of your microbes are very much invested in your well-being. If you die, they die, too, and when you prosper, so do they. It is the ultimate symbiotic relationship, and when it's healthy and well maintained, both you and your microbes thrive.

We can categorize your microscopic roommates into three main groups:

1. Commensal bacteria that cohabit peacefully with you, like *Streptococcus salivarius* in your mouth that are simply part of your normal bacterial ecosystem.

2. Symbiotic organisms (sometimes called mutualists) that play an active role in keeping you healthy, like certain strains of *Escherichia coli* in the gut that synthesize vitamin K, which is required for your blood to be able to clot properly.
3. Pathogens (including opportunistic flora) that can do you harm, like *Pseudomonas aeruginosa,* which can cause ear infections.

In a balanced healthy microbiome, groups 1 and 2, the quintessential "good" bacteria, far outnumber the pathogens or "bad" bacteria. There's no requirement for a microbiome composed entirely of good bacteria, but without sufficient commensals and symbiotic species, your microbiome can't function properly—and neither can the rest of your body, particularly your immune system.

TABLE 1.1 • Predominant Bacteria Present in Humans

LOCATION	BACTERIA
Skin	*Staphylococci, Corynebacteria*
Mouth	*Streptococci, Lactobacilli*
Nose	*Staphylococci, Corynebacteria*
Throat	*Streptococci, Neisseria*
Stomach	*Helicobacter pylori*
Small intestine	*Bifidobacteria, Enterococci*
Colon	*Bacteroides, Enterococci, Clostridia*
Urinary tract	*Corynebacteria*
Vagina	*Lactic acid bacteria*

What Do Your Gut Bacteria Do?

Symbiotic organisms—the quintessential "good" bacteria—perform lots of important functions. They help you digest food, maintain the integrity of your gut lining (the barrier that keeps bowel contents—and viruses—separate from the rest of your body), crowd out harmful pathogens, and train your immune system to distinguish between friend and foe. They also convert carbohydrates into critical metabolites like short-chain fatty acids (SCFAs) that help guide your immune response, and they synthesize many of the enzymes, vitamins, and hormones that you can't make on your own. Food can't be properly broken down and its constituent parts can't be fully absorbed without these essential gut bacteria, which means that even if you're eating a super-nutritious diet, if you don't have a healthy microbiome, you may not be able to absorb and assimilate all of the vitamins and nutrients in your food.

ROLE OF GUT MICROBES
- Digest food
- Produce digestive enzymes
- Convert carbohydrates to short-chain fatty acids (SCFAs)
- Help your body absorb nutrients such as calcium and iron
- Synthesize B-complex vitamins like thiamine and folate
- Synthesize fat-soluble vitamins like vitamin K
- Synthesize hormones and neurotransmitters
- Maintain the integrity of the gut lining
- Keep the pH in your gut balanced
- Metabolize drugs
- Neutralize cancer-causing compounds
- Promote angiogenesis (growth of new blood vessels)
- Crowd out pathogens
- Train the immune system to distinguish friend from foe
- Activate anti-viral efforts
- Modulate genes

You're Only as Healthy as Your Gut Bacteria

Ever notice how some people never get sick when everyone else has the flu or a cold? They're exposed to the same virus as everyone else, but because of their healthy microbiome populated with lots of essential "good" microbes, they're able to defeat the virus and stay healthy. The very young, whose microbiome is still developing and who therefore lack the microbial diversity necessary for a strong immune system, and the very old, who also have fewer microbial species and less diversity, tend to be the most vulnerable, but there are lots of external factors at play, too, in which we have a key role. The medications we take, the food we choose to put on our plates every day, and the environments we expose ourselves to are some of the major influences that we have control over. Overzealous use of antibiotics can put you at risk for viral infection by killing off good microbes along with the bad ones; a low-fiber diet literally starves many of the bacterial species that are essential for proper immune function; and a super-sanitized environment can also put us at risk by exposing us to pesticides and other microbe-depleting chemicals and limiting our contact with soil microbes that can enhance our own internal bacterial communities. (I'll get much more into the nitty-gritty of these enemies of the microbiome in Chapter 11.)

. . . . .

Now that you have a better sense of your microbiome and the many important functions it performs throughout your body, let's focus on how your gut microbes and your immune system are connected and how that relationship, when it's healthy, protects you from viruses.

HAND IN GLOVE

Your body is in constant contact with external and internal threats that pose a direct danger to your health: harmful viruses and other pathogens in the environment, plus internal waste and toxins that can build up in your body and lead to chronic inflammation and disease. Your immune system protects you from all of it—cancer, infection, and more—and helps you recover after injury. It's your first and best line of defense, and it's especially important now, with the reality of global pandemics, plus all the chemicals and carcinogens we're exposed to on a daily basis. But how does this internal surveillance system actually work to protect you from viruses? It turns out that your gut microbiome and your immune system have an extremely close interdependent relationship, and that hand in glove interaction is critical to a properly functioning immune system that can keep you safe and healthy.

Your immune system tolerates an enormous and constantly changing mass of harmless microbes, while at the same time recognizing and responding to dangerous viruses that it's able to spot amid a pool of trillions of other organisms. How is it able to distinguish friend from foe so precisely and then launch an attack that destroys one while preserving the other? The fact that more than 70 percent of your immune system is located in your gut provides an important clue. The thin lining of your intestinal wall, known as your epithelial barrier, has immune cells on one side and bacteria on the other, and both sides interact continuously with each other. Immune cells in your gut lining pump out substances to help defend against invaders, while microbes help guide and modulate those cells, ensuring a balanced immune response. Let's go over some immunology basics to better understand the relationship.

Immunology 101

Your immune system is made up of two armies: an innate system that you're born with and an adaptive one that develops over time. Your innate system is your body's first line of defense, responding quickly but in a general and nonspecific way to invading pathogens. For instance, if you get a cut in your skin, your innate immune system activates cells and proteins that kill any bacteria that may have entered through the wound.

Adaptive immunity takes longer to develop because it evolves from learned experiences. It keeps a record of every potential pathogen you've encountered, so that it can recognize and destroy the pathogen when it enters your body again, utilizing more precise weaponry that targets the specific germ you're trying to fend off. While it may take a few days for adaptive immunity to kick in the first time you encounter a virus, the next exposure will generally result in a much faster response, and for some viruses, like measles, no illness at all with subsequent encounters because you have become "immune." Vaccines rely on adaptive immunity: when a small, harmless amount of protein from a virus is introduced into your body, your adaptive immune system will remember it if and when it encounters it again. Adaptive immunity is also known as acquired immunity and involves two different types of white blood cells: B lymphocytes, which make antibodies that destroy the pathogen itself, and T lymphocytes, which act as air traffic control for your immune system—removing any cells that have been infected and damaged by the pathogen, activating other immune cells, and regulating the immune response.

For some infections, like the flu, adaptive immunity doesn't reliably protect you because there are lots of different viruses or strains, and catching a cold or flu from one doesn't usually provide specific immunity against others. As we've seen with SARS-CoV-2, viruses can also mutate, and the new variant may not be recognizable to your adaptive immune system. Sometimes there can be overlap, though, and an infection with one virus can give you some protection against another. That's what researchers in Boston found when they identified people who had previously been infected with harmless coronavirus variants. When those same people got infected with SARS-CoV-2 years later, they weren't as sick. They had lower rates of needing a ventilator, fewer ICU admissions, and fewer deaths. Those Boston patients were a classic example of how prior exposure to germs can actually prime your immune system so that it can protect you from more dangerous pathogens down the road.

Another example of protective adaptive immunity was seen with the 2009 H1N1 influenza strain. When it emerged, it caused more severe illness in younger people. Globally, four out of five H1N1 deaths occurred in people under sixty-five. That's very atypical for flu deaths, which usually occur in older adults. It turned out that many of the older people had been exposed to a relative of the strain decades ago—and that previous exposure created a memory within their immune system that was able to protect them from H1N1.

Too Much

Having good adaptive immunity is one thing, but a stronger than normal immune response can actually lead to problems. Too much or too prolonged an immune response can create overreaction to common exposures and cause food allergies, reactions to medications, allergies to bee or wasp stings, asthma, hay fever (allergic rhinitis), hives (urticaria), and dermatitis. These are all conditions that have become commonplace in the last half century and directly correlate with abnormalities in our microbiome that have also occurred during this time period. One example is the startling increase in the incidence and severity of food allergies, which coincides with an increasingly processed food supply and high antibiotic use.

Autoimmune diseases, a family of chronic, often debilitating, and in some cases life-threatening illnesses that affect almost one in five Americans, are another classic example of an overactive immune system. Their mechanism, regardless of what organ they affect, is that they prompt your immune system to wage war against your body's own healthy tissues, overreacting to normal stimuli with an exaggerated inflammatory response. Autoimmune diseases represent a new breed of illness that emerged mostly in the last century and include conditions like Hashimoto's thyroiditis, type 1 diabetes, lupus, multiple sclerosis (MS), rheumatoid arthritis, inflammatory bowel disease (Crohn's and ulcerative colitis), eczema, and psoriasis. There are more than a hundred different types of autoimmune diseases, and chances are you or someone in your family suffers from one (or more) since they affect about fifty million people in the United States alone. Different autoimmune diseases frequently affect the same person, suggesting a common root cause with varied manifestations rather than multiple distinct illnesses. In addition to genetic predisposition, depletion of good bacteria from antibiotics and other medications, as well as a diet that's lacking in the fiber needed to support the growth of essential species, are at the root of many autoimmune diseases.

Not Enough

An underactive immune system (immunodeficiency) means your immune system's ability to fight infections as well as most types of cancer is compromised or entirely absent. Most cases are acquired ("secondary") due to illnesses like HIV infection or environmental factors like malnutrition. Immunodeficiency can also be due to genetic diseases that you're born with ("primary"), like severe combined immunodeficiency (SCID). Another common cause of immunodeficiency is medications that weaken your immune system, like biologics, steroids, or chemotherapy. Not only do these drugs dramatically increase your risk of infection—especially infections from viruses as well as "opportunistic" organisms that in immunocompetent people are usually benign and harmless—but they also interfere with your immune system's ability to detect and remove malignant cells, putting you at increased risk for cancer, too.

Just Right

Successfully fighting viral infections relies on what I like to call the Goldilocks principle: an immune response that's strong enough to clear the virus and keep you safe, but not so powerful that it damages parts of your body and harms you in the process—a condition known as cytokine storm. And this is where having a healthy gut comes in, since your gut bacteria are intimately involved in guiding your immune system to create that immune equilibrium. How exactly does it do that?

ANTI-VIRAL STRATEGIES

Mice raised experimentally without a microbiome can't survive in the real world outside of a sterile environment—and neither can germ-free humans. Bacteria in your gut are involved in every step of your immune response and employ specific strategies to protect you from viral infections.

The most important way your gut bacteria protect you is by regulating your immune system to make sure you have the appropriate response when you encounter a virus. Since most of your immune system is in your digestive tract, it's not surprising that your immune response is heavily influenced by the number and diversity of your microbes. Gut bacteria train your immune system how and when to respond to threats, turning up the response to fight invading viruses, or turning it down in situations where overshooting the mark and recruiting too many immune cells could lead to excess inflammation and organ damage—the deadly cytokine storm we've become so familiar with during the COVID pandemic. An intact and healthy complement of gut bacteria is therefore not only beneficial but also necessary for that Goldilocks immune equilibrium: a response that's robust enough to clear viruses but not so active that it ends up doing more harm than good.

Another anti-viral strategy of gut bacteria is creating a physical barrier that blocks viruses from penetrating deeper into your body. Viruses literally have to wade through a dense army of bacteria—plus their surrounding web of mucus and the epithelial gut lining—to penetrate common entry points like your nose, mouth, gastrointestinal tract, and lungs. A compromised microbiome weakens that physical barrier, creating cracks that allow viruses to seep through, gain access to your internal organs, and run amok in your body.

Deploying chemical weapons against viruses is another way your microbes protect you. When confronted with a viral threat, gut bacteria trigger your immune cells to release virus-repelling substances called interferons (so named because they "interfere" with viruses and keep them from multiplying). Interferons are proteins that are part of your natural artillery against viruses. They notify your immune system when harmful germs or cancer cells are in your body, and they recruit killer immune cells to fight those invaders. Common gut bacteria like *Bacteroides fragilis* and other commensals in your digestive system are the ones that raise the alarm and stimulate immune cells in the walls of your intestines to release interferons and other chemical weapons.

Here's an example of how it works: The very contagious rotavirus causes a diarrheal illness that kills half a million children each year. But when anti-viral proteins from specific gut bacteria are injected into mice suffering from rotavirus, they successfully halt the infection. Not surprisingly, we see almost five times higher rates of rotavirus and more severe infection in children who have recently been treated with antibiotics and are missing some of those crucial protective bacteria. The same mechanism of bacterial protection is also true for other viruses like influenza, with increased susceptibility and worse symptoms when antibiotics precede the viral illness.

In order for viruses to infect a cell, they need to attach to specific receptor sites (also called binding sites) on the cell membrane. They accomplish this through special attachment proteins in their protective shell that surround the virus's genetic material. In the case of SARS-CoV-2, those now famous spike proteins bind to ACE-2 receptors that predominate in our lungs and gastrointestinal (GI) tract. The ability of a virus to attach to a specific receptor determines what cells it can infect, which is why we see so many respiratory and GI symptoms with COVID. Bacteria like *Lactobacillus* outsmart viruses like coronavirus by competing for the same binding sites, which interferes with the ability of the virus to bind to their receptors. Without that binding, the virus can't enter cells in your body and cause illness. And that's why we need lots of helpful bacteria like *Lactobacillus* around.

Predictive Power

Infection with a virus prompts your immune system to produce substances (cytokines) that control the growth and activity of other immune cells and help manage the immune response. In some cases, this response can be excessive, causing widespread tissue damage, septic shock, and multiorgan failure. This so-called cytokine storm is a leading cause of death in people with severe cases of COVID. Analysis of these patients shows that underlying microbial imbalance is associated with elevated levels of inflammatory cytokines and tissue damage, confirming the influence of the microbiome on the immune system response.

People with severe viral infections often lack certain helpful bacterial species in their gut that are essential for regulating their immune response. The resulting immune disequilibrium as a result of those missing microbes is what puts you at risk for life-threatening inflammation, not just in your lungs but throughout your body. In a large study of patients with COVID, the composition of the microbiome predicted development of severe respiratory symptoms and death with 92 percent accuracy, which is much more accurate than cardiovascular status, age, or other traditional assessments of outcome. Why is this so important? Because unlike your genes, which are fairly static, or your age, which you can't change, or heart disease, which you may not be able to reverse, you have a great deal of control over what's going on in your gut. The purpose of this book is to help you connect the dots between your gut health and your immune health and chart a course to make sure both are fully optimized to protect you.

If we take a closer look at the digestive system of COVID patients with poor outcomes, we see high levels of an undesirable gut bacteria called *Enterococcus faecalis* (*E. faecalis*). *E. faecalis* can penetrate your gut lining, enter your bloodstream, and cause life-threatening infection, and that's why overrepresentation of *E. faecalis* in your microbiome is so dangerous. High levels of this bacteria are the top predictor of COVID severity. But just as too much of an undesirable species like *E. faecalis* can be problematic, not enough helpful ones can be just as deadly. Disease severity in COVID is inversely correlated with the gut bacteria *Faecalibacterium prausnitzii* (*F. prausnitzii*)—an essential and highly beneficial species that's cultivated by eating a high-fiber diet. The relationship between *F. prausnitzii* and viral infections is clear and direct: the more *F. prausnitzii* in your gut, the less sick you'll be if you get infected.

If you're trying to predict who is going to do well and who is at serious risk during a viral outbreak, you need look no further than the gut. A small smear of stool obtained from your rectum will provide you with more valuable and accurate information than any other data points, including demographic information like age, ethnicity, or gender; clinical data like oxygen saturation, inflammatory markers, or levels of white blood cells; or medical history like whether you have heart disease, diabetes, or lung disease. Even when you combine all of these factors, they still don't have the predictive power that assessing the health of your microbiome does, and that's true not just for COVID but for almost any viral infection. In the future, as we learn even more about which species help versus hinder, microbiome assessment may become a vital tool in identifying at-risk groups who need earlier intervention or closer monitoring when infected.

We know that compared to healthy people, people who get sick from viral infections tend to have preexisting conditions like obesity, cardiovascular disease, diabetes, or a weakened immune system, but all of these conditions are themselves strongly correlated with an unhealthy microbiome. Given what we know about the connection between the health of your microbiome and outcomes from viruses, it's not surprising that these patients are sicker. But why do so many people have an unhealthy microbiome in the first place? What is it about our current lifestyle that creates changes in our gut flora that put us at risk?

In Praise of Germs

Modern practices such as chlorinated drinking water, industrial agriculture, pesticides, and antibiotics have improved our lives in countless ways, but they've also brought health challenges by creating a super-sanitized environment that's associated with less microbial richness and diversity. Alcohol and the high-fat/high-sugar highly processed Western diet compound the problem because they don't nourish our essential gut flora. That leads to a decrease in important bacterial metabolites that are necessary for immune equilibrium and an increased risk of autoimmune diseases, allergies, and more severe viral infections.

You need interaction with germs to train your immune system how to respond appropriately to stimuli in your environment—what to react to and what to ignore. An immune system that doesn't get up close and personal with enough germs early on is like a child with overprotective parents—ill-equipped to deal with problems when they inevitably happen. Not having enough exposure to microbes can lead to defects in your immune tolerance, which means a trigger-happy state of heightened activity where harmless encounters with normal gut bacteria, proteins in food, and even parts of your own body are treated like the enemy and attacked by your immune system.

Of course, during a pandemic a certain level of vigilance about exposure to germs is required. The trick is to employ tactics that rid your immediate surroundings of any viral threats while still maintaining exposure to health-promoting microbes. You also need to feed your gut bacteria an appropriate diet so they can churn out substances to help protect you, and avoid unnecessary antimicrobials that are ruinous to your bacterial foot soldiers. I'll provide all the details about how to do this in Part 3, "Strengthening from Within—the Anti-Viral Gut Plan." In the meantime, let me tell you about one of my patients who was fortunate to have lots of exposure to nature, microbes, and fibrous vegetables growing up, and what happened when that all changed.

THE MICROBIOME-LIFESTYLE CONNECTION

I diagnosed a patient of mine, Anjali (you may remember her if you read my second book, *The Microbiome Solution*), with Crohn's disease two years after she moved to the United States from India to attend college. She was raised in a vegetarian household in a village where every day, her mother or one of her relatives cooked lentils, chickpeas, mung beans, potatoes, okra, and other locally grown vegetables from scratch, made with plenty of anti-inflammatory spices like turmeric, and shared by multiple generations of her extended family living together in the same household. When she moved to the United States, Anjali continued to eat a vegetarian diet, but one that looked very different from what she grew up on: her daily fare was now pizza, french fries, bagels, and the contents of the vending machines at school. She developed adult acne, acid reflux, and indigestion that eventually turned into bloody diarrhea and severe ulceration throughout most of her colon and small intestine.

Anjali had never heard of Crohn's disease and didn't know anyone who had it, but her case was one of the most severe I had ever diagnosed. We eventually got her into remission using a combination of conventional medication and dietary modification, reinstituting an unprocessed high-fiber diet similar to what she ate as a child in India. In her case, it seemed that the protective effect of growing up in a rural environment with lots of exposure to microbes and fibrous foods was no match for the detrimental effects of the Western diet and a super-sanitized lifestyle. Anjali's story illustrates the importance of a healthy microbiome in protecting you against disease, especially those that involve your immune system.

It's What's Inside That Really Counts

When I hear reports of people having severe COVID, or worse, even succumbing to the virus, in addition to feeling sad for their families and loved ones, I'm always immensely curious about their medical history—particularly what's going on in their gut. Someone may look perfectly fine on the outside, but do they have a healthy-functioning immune system? Are they dealing with an autoimmune disease that puts them at high risk for poor outcomes as a result of a disordered microbiome? Have they been on medication that may have significantly altered their gut flora? What does their diet look like? There are lots of additional determinants of health that play a role in outcome from viral infection—and we'll be discussing several of them throughout this book—but the gut-immune connection is fundamental to your ability to survive and thrive in a world full of viruses. To understand the significance of gut and immune health in the context of viral threats, it's helpful to introduce another concept that is as consequential as germ theory, if not more so.

Your Terrain

Around the same time Pasteur was popularizing his theory, another Frenchman, Antoine Béchamp, proposed an alternative view of how and why we get sick. Béchamp's "terrain theory" stated that disease isn't able to develop in a truly healthy environment and that germs lead to disease only in an unhealthy host. Put another way, terrain theory focuses on the soil rather than the seed and makes the case that the same pathogen ("seed") can pass harmlessly through your body rather than make you sick if your ecosystem ("soil") is healthy. Therefore, paying attention to the health of the host, elements like our microbiome and immune system that make up our "terrain"—not just the potency of the pathogen we're confronted with—creates resilience to a wide range of infections and illnesses. Béchamp believed that the more unhealthy and out of balance you are, the more susceptible you are to illness and the sicker you'll get when you come into contact with a virus.

As physicians, we see germ theory at work every day when people become ill after exposure to specific pathogens. But it's also logical that our body's terrain is a powerful force in helping to protect us against those illnesses. Terrain theory suggests that if a person has a healthy and well-balanced microbiome and immune system, any organisms they encounter will be dealt with by their body without causing severe sickness. Both theories play an important role in understanding how exposure to viruses can lead to illness.

We wash our hands and avoid people who are sick because of germ theory, but we maintain a well-functioning ecosystem that's able to fight viruses through eating a healthy diet and minimizing exposure to immune-suppressing and microbe-depleting drugs because of terrain theory. The realization that the health of the host, not just the potency of the pathogen, also determines the outcome from viral exposure is a simple but essential concept. Once you understand that you, as the host, are in the driver's seat when it comes to battling viruses, the path forward for how to emerge victorious becomes clear.

Overkill

Treating an off-kilter terrain with heavy hitters like immune-suppressing drugs or broad-spectrum antibiotics is like using Roundup to get rid of a few weeds in your backyard. It will definitely destroy any problematic giant hogweed or poison ivy, but at great cost to the insects and soil microbes that are the foundation of any healthy garden. Adrian Higgins, a former *Washington Post* columnist and the author of three garden books, thinks that if you are turning to herbicides regularly, there is something wrong with your approach to gardening. I think the same can be said of an entirely medicalized approach to restoring or maintaining health that doesn't take into account the important nutritional and lifestyle factors that are at the heart of gut and immune well-being. When you prescribe steroids for autoimmune disease, or doxycycline for acne, you are treating a symptom, not the problem. Of course medications aren't the only thing that mess up your terrain—as I'll explain in Part 2, the Standard American Diet, too much stress, not enough sleep, and a number of other factors also compromise the health of your soil.

Weeds fill empty spaces and thrive in disturbed soil. If you spray them without addressing the void, they return swiftly. So the most effective and sustainable way to control them is to crowd them out with beneficial plants. I'm not a gardener, but as an integrative gastroenterologist, I advocate a microbe-sparing approach to illness whenever possible, for the simple reason that repopulation yields healthier crops—and guts—than eradication. For example, in my patients with bacterial overgrowth, instead of antibiotics I recommend restoring their terrain with fermented foods, a high-fiber diet, select probiotics, and daily exposure to dirt. It takes a little longer to work but has a high rate of success, has a low likelihood of recurrence, doesn't remove large swaths of healthy bacteria along with whatever you're trying to eradicate, and avoids secondary problems like yeast overgrowth that antibiotics cause. These are the benefits of a terrain-restoring approach.

FORENSICS

We hear about "totally healthy" people succumbing to viral infections all the time. While that can and does happen, diseases, including viral ones, generally don't just fall out of the sky and flatten us. We can almost always, according to principles of science and logic, predictably follow the breadcrumbs backward to uncover the vulnerability in our terrain that allowed infection and illness to develop.

Understanding the importance of your own innate host defenses and appreciating how easily they can be dismantled provides an opportunity to think about prevention in new ways that are less scorched earth, more organic gardening, and ultimately more successful.

GETTING SICK IS NOT INEVITABLE

Exposure to viruses on its own isn't what makes us sick; it's defects in our terrain—depletion of our healthy gut bacteria, an imbalanced immune response, our stressed-out modern lifestyle, and an ultra-processed diet—that ultimately turn that exposure into an illness. Exposure to viruses is inevitable. Getting sick is not. Sometimes you're dealing with a really bad bug, and no matter what you do, you're screwed. But more often than not, a defect in your terrain is what turns that exposure into a winner for the virus and causes you to lose the battle.

The health of the host is as important as the potency of the pathogen—maybe even more important. We need an intact and well-functioning microbiome and immune system in order to make sure that inevitable encounters with viruses don't lead to serious infection. But what if I told you that not all viruses pose a threat to your health and that in fact many of the astonishingly large number of them living inside you form part of your genetic makeup and play a role in keeping you—and the planet—alive? In the next chapter we'll explore the fascinating and only recently discovered world of the virome and its relationship to human health.

To view the scientific references cited in this chapter, please visit
drrobynnechutkan.com/anti-viral-gut-references.

2

Welcome to the Virome

If all viruses suddenly disappeared, the world would be a wonderful place for about a day and a half, and then we'd all die.
— Tony Goldberg, PhD, Professor of Epidemiology

A decade ago we were barely aware of the community of viruses that live inside us. Today we know the human virome is an integral part of our microbiome—the immense ecosystem of microscopic organisms that inhabit our bodies—and the more we learn about the virome, the more we realize it's a partnership that can affect us both positively and negatively. Viruses fall into the same categories of "good" and "bad" that we use to categorize the bacteria that cohabitate with us, and contrary to what you might think based on recent events, harmful viruses are actually in the minority compared to benign ones. Some of the viruses that inhabit your body can cause illness, but the majority coexist peacefully with you, and some actually protect you. Just as only a few species of bacteria are truly dangerous, the vast majority of viruses are not harmful to humans. And like bacteria, viruses also play a key role in maintaining our health—and the health of the planet. Let's find out more about these unusual organisms that are completely dependent on their hosts for their life and livelihood.

VIRUSES ARE EVERYWHERE

This pandemic has forced a little virology on all of us, and since viruses are an increasingly relevant part of our world, it's important to understand some basics. The first thing you should know is that your body is brimming with them. You have ten times as many bacterial cells as human cells, and ten times as many viruses as bacteria. How many viruses is that? About 380 trillion (more than stars in the universe!). But viruses aren't just in your body, they're also everywhere in the environment, from the Sahara Desert to the oceans, with more than a million in a single drop of seawater. As you'll discover in this chapter, despite the recent bad rap, viruses are way more good than they are bad—not just for us, but also for the planet.

PART OF US

In order to survive and replicate, viruses have to infect a living bacterial, animal, or plant cell. On its own, a virus is just genetic material surrounded by a protective protein shell. But once it gets into your body, it comes to life, hijacking your cells for its own life cycle purposes and even incorporating its genetic material into your genes and becoming part of your DNA. When a virus, whether a benign or virulent one, encounters a host cell, it attaches itself to the wall of the cell, enters, travels to the cell's genetic material, merges with its genes, and then tricks the host's genetic machinery into making copies of itself. If it happens to infect an egg or sperm cell, the virus's genetic material becomes inserted into that cell's genetic code and can be passed down to subsequent generations. As a result, as much as 10 percent of our genetic material is actually made up of bits of viral DNA that have gradually become part of our genes. These viral remnants in our genetic code are involved in some of our most important bodily functions, including encoding memories and making placental proteins involved in human reproduction—examples of how viruses serve an important role in our own evolution.

JUST TRYING TO SURVIVE

Viruses can be scary, but they don't have evil murderous intentions— they're just trying to find a host to inhabit so they can survive. When you're exposed to a relatively new virus, your immune system doesn't recognize it as a threat because it's never seen it before, and so it allows it to enter your body. But once that virus starts to infect your cells, your immune system kicks into gear by releasing chemicals to try to wipe out the viral invaders. This immune-mediated attack may end up making you feel sick, but those symptoms are mostly a result of your immune system fighting back. Here are some of the symptoms you may experience with a viral infection that are actually signs of your body trying to get rid of the virus:

TABLE 2.1 • Making Sense of Your Viral Symptoms

SYMPTOM	PURPOSE
Runny nose/nasal congestion	Washes virus particles out of your nose and sinuses
Coughing and sneezing	Traps virus in mucus, then expels it from your body
Fever	Destroys viruses, which are heat sensitive and can't survive high temperatures
Muscle aches and pain	Pulls protein from your muscles to help fight the virus, causing aches and soreness

Some of your body's virus-fighting responses can actually help spread the virus, like coughing and sneezing, which disperse viral particles out into the environment, where they can be inhaled by other potential hosts. As your immune system literally turns up the heat with fever and other tactics designed to get rid of it, the virus needs to find some way of spreading to other hosts in order to survive. Natural selection provides a number of strategies for pathogens to make that leap, including:

TABLE 2.2 • Virus Spreading Tactics (Going Viral—Literally!)

TRANSMISSION	DISEASE	TACTIC
Droplet	Influenza	Infection gets transmitted when you sneeze on someone
Airborne	SARS-CoV-2	Infectious particles get exhaled by you and inhaled by someone else
Vector	West Nile	Pathogen gets transmitted from you to another host by a vector carrier, like a mosquito
Waterborne	Rotavirus	Infected feces get into the water supply and spread the infection to others when they drink the contaminated water
Sit-and-wait	Herpes Simplex	Organism stays dormant for a long time (sometimes years) and then reactivates once it comes into contact with a new host

A DELICATE BALANCE: TRANSMISSION VERSUS VIRULENCE

Have you ever wondered why some viruses are deadly enough to kill you, while others just give you the sniffles? As we discussed in the previous chapter, your terrain (microbiome and immune system) is a major contributor to the outcome after a viral exposure and one that's determined solely by you, the host. But there are additional factors that affect outcome that are determined by the virus, not the host, and some of those variables involve an important trade-off that viruses have to make between virulence and transmission.

For viruses, transmission is a matter of life or death, and that means they have to pay attention to what they're doing to you, the host. If a virus is super virulent and replicates too quickly, it will make lots of viral copies, but it may also kill you off before its offspring have an opportunity to find a new home. If it does less harm and replicates slowly, it won't generate as many viral offspring, but it may increase its chances of spreading because you'll be healthy and more likely to interact with others and spread the virus. Natural selection balances this evolutionary trade-off between virulence and transmission, selecting for pathogens virulent enough to produce many offspring that can infect new hosts, but not so virulent that they kill off the original host before it can help with transmission. This is important to keep in mind because it helps inform our strategies when confronted with viral threats, particularly new ones.

OLDIE VERSUS NEWBIE VIRUSES

Viruses that have been around for a while (like the measles virus, which appeared about four thousand years ago) have had lots of time to figure out that they need to keep you alive so you can help them spread, so they tend to make you less sick. Over the many years they've been around, they've figured out that killing you also puts them at risk of becoming extinct. Their evolutionary need to find new hosts can lead to symptoms like coughing and sneezing, which increase the likelihood of your dispersing them to others while still keeping you relatively healthy.

Newer viruses that aren't yet well adapted to humans can be much more deadly, like Ebola, which has a fatality rate of over 50 percent. Instead of peaceful coexistence, Ebola's survival strategy is to replicate rapidly, infect all your tissues, and turn you into a puddle of infectious virus particles in the hopes that your bodily fluids will drip onto someone else and infect them. What that means for us, as potential hosts, is that we have to adjust our anti-viral strategies and tactics based on what we know about a virus's virulence and transmission. A high-fatality-rate virus that's über-transmissible will necessitate a very different playbook of anti-viral behavior compared to one with a less than 2 percent fatality rate, like we've seen with SARS-CoV-2.

THE UPSIDE

Despite our focused efforts on decreasing transmission, it's important to realize that viral infection isn't always a bad thing. While you may view it as a purely negative experience, chronic viral infection may actually provide you with immune benefits and decrease your susceptibility to other diseases. Certain strains of redondovirus found in the lungs, for example, are involved in helping you fight respiratory illnesses, and enzymes from some viruses can kill antibiotic-resistant strains of harmful bacteria. A virus similar to the one that causes dengue fever is linked to delayed progression to AIDS in HIV-positive people. Infection with herpes virus can provide some unexpected advantages that probably evolved over time to help us survive past threats: both mice and humans infected with herpes are less susceptible to bubonic plague.

While it's important to have a strong and effective anti-viral gut, it's equally important to understand that the goal is balance and not indiscriminate eradication of all viruses.

Fortunately, our gut-based immune system is pretty good at distinguishing between viruses that pose a threat to us and those that are a benign—or even helpful—part of our microscopic community. Once that determination is made, there are some pretty slick additional gut-based defenses that spring into action to rid your body of problematic viruses. Some consist of changes in the physical environment within your body to make things less hospitable for the viral invaders, while others involve actual entrapment and expulsion of viruses. We'll find out more about these critical anti-viral gut weapons in the next chapter.

To view the scientific references cited in this chapter, please visit

drrobynnechutkan.com/anti-viral-gut-references.

3

Host Defenses

*What seems insignificant when you have it, is important when you
need it.*

—Franz Grillparzer

Your body almost always has your back. If you've been overdoing
it at the gym, pain from an overworked muscle will force you to
take a break so it can heal. Thank goodness for hangovers or we'd
probably all die from alcohol poisoning (especially during a pandemic!). I remind my patients that heartburn after a late-night pizza
binge isn't a disease, just their sleepy stomachs reminding them that
two a.m. isn't the ideal time to digest food. The helpful feedback your
body gives you isn't always negative: that well-rested take-on-the-
world feeling you have after a great night's sleep can make you want
to do it again, and endorphins released when you exercise can be really motivating and help you reach your workout goals. But whether
it's a negative "that probably wasn't such a good idea" reminder, or a
positive "wow, I should definitely do that again" nudge, your body's
feedback usually moves you in the direction of better health, and ig-
noring or suppressing it can have unexpected negative consequences.

In this chapter, I'll show you that in addition to your immune system, your gut has some additional tricks up its sleeve to keep you safe

from viruses. Much like the swimmer at the beach who is blissfully unaware of the great white shark swimming a few feet away, most of the time you have no idea about the catastrophe that could have—but didn't—happen, thanks to your amazing anti-viral gut defenses. And it's interfering with these protective mechanisms, not randomness and bad luck, that often leads to poor outcomes from viral encounters. If you want to ensure you're on the winning end of the battle against a virus, it's critical to understand how those defenses work to protect you, and to question practices and prescriptions that may sabotage them.

ACID

For nearly 600 people sickened during a Royal Caribbean cruise to the Caribbean, their vacation was no day at the beach. About a fifth of the 3,050 people aboard *Explorer of the Seas,* which left Cape Liberty, New Jersey, for a ten-day cruise in January 2014, came down with an illness.

People were vomiting into bags, into buckets, or on the floor of the ship's infirmary. The 50 percent refund and additional 50 percent future cruise credit seemed like chump change compensation for the days of misery holed up in cabins with stomach cramps, vomiting, diarrhea, and malaise.

That norovirus episode was, at the time, the largest viral outbreak ever reported on a cruise ship, with one in five aboard coming down with the highly contagious virus, which spreads by contact with infected people, contaminated food, water, or surfaces. There are more than twenty million cases of norovirus every year in the United States (only the common cold is more frequent), and as is true with most viruses, its sweet spot is small spaces with lots of people.

But here's the conundrum: common areas in cruise ships are

crowded, so when hundreds of people are spewing gazillions of highly contagious viral particles everywhere and contaminating most of the surfaces, why do only a fraction of the other passengers get sick? The average stateroom on a ship is about the size of a master bathroom, but even for two people sleeping together in the same small cabin, it's not uncommon for one person to become infected while the other one doesn't.

Clearly, exposure alone doesn't tell the whole story. Certain people just seem to be more susceptible to viruses. The immune system is waxing in the very young and waning in the very old, so it makes sense that extremes of age make you more vulnerable. So does taking immunosuppressive drugs that interfere with your body's ability to fight infection, or having a lot of chronic medical problems that make you frailer and less able to defend yourself from viral attack. But beyond those well-documented risk factors, is there something that healthy people are doing every day that may be sabotaging one of their critical host defenses and greatly increasing their likelihood of picking up a virus? It turns out that taking commonly prescribed acid blockers could be the culprit, but why?

Why Stomach Acid Is a Good Thing

Acid is essential for digestion—that's why your stomach makes it! Stomach acid activates an enzyme called pepsin, which breaks proteins down into amino acids that your body can absorb, and it's also necessary for absorption of vitamin B_{12} and other important nutrients that can be properly assimilated only in an acidic environment. The release of stomach acid produces chemical signals that stimulate other digestive organs, like the pancreas, and it triggers peristalsis, the muscular contractions of the intestines that help mix and move the products of digestion through the rest of the gastrointestinal (GI) tract. Stomach acid also helps prevent food poisoning because potentially harmful microbes in your food and drink can't survive in an acidic environment.

The Benefits and Costs of PPIs

If you've ever been to see a gastroenterologist or complained to your internist about any sort of heartburn, indigestion, or abdominal discomfort, chances are they've either written you a prescription for an acid-blocking medication or recommended that you buy an over-the-counter version of one. Acid blockers have been popularized and mass marketed to the public in advertisements that show people comfortably tucking into a late-night cheeseburger or gobbling down an entire pepperoni pizza without so much as a whisper of complaint from their digestive tract. They're among the top ten most prescribed drugs in the world, with estimated annual sales of $14 billion, because they're really, really good at what they do, which is to completely shut down the acid pump in your stomach. I'm talking specifically about the class of acid-blocking drugs known as proton pump inhibitors (PPIs).

Given the central role that stomach acid plays in digestion, it's not surprising that blocking it leads to all sorts of problems: incomplete digestion and decreased absorption of nutrients and fat-soluble vitamins that require acid for proper assimilation, and an increase in foodborne illnesses. Interference with digestion and absorption is behind most of the long-term side effects of PPIs, including bone fractures, kidney disease, and anemia. Perhaps the most problematic side effect, though, is how these drugs make you more vulnerable to infection.

Here's how that works: when you turn off acid production, you transform your stomach from an inhospitable acidic environment that kills viruses by denaturing and inactivating their proteins, to a friendly breeding ground where viruses can flourish and thrive because all the acid has been removed and the pH is now alkaline, which is safe for viruses. Simply put, stomach acid kills pathogens. Not having any may improve your reflux symptoms, but it leaves you particularly vulnerable to viral invasion and infection of your intestinal cells, which is one of the main ways viruses enter your body. Stomach acid is one of your most important and effective host defenses, and without it, you're much more vulnerable to viruses. A lack of stomach acid is what's behind the dramatically increased risk of viral infections we see in people taking PPIs, and that's well illustrated on cruise ship outbreaks where the average passenger is between forty-five and sixty—an age group with high PPI usage.

By reducing the acid load in your stomach, PPIs don't just remove your stomach's ability to kill viruses, they also promote overgrowth of the wrong type of bacteria in your upper gastrointestinal tract, because the highly acidic state that would normally curtail growth is no longer in effect. That disrupts the natural balance of your microbiome, not unlike the effects of antibiotics—and makes it easier for pathogens to flourish. That unchecked growth of pathogens caused by PPIs is linked to viral pneumonia, as well as gut-related viral infections. PPIs also promote pneumonia by suppressing coughing, a frequent symptom of reflux that helps prevent acid from traveling up into your airway and serves the dual purpose of clearing pathogens from your lungs. Yes—stomach acid is a really important host defense!

The Real Price of PPIs

When used judiciously for short periods of time for bleeding ulcers, or chronically for precancerous esophageal changes (Barrett's esophagus) or severe inflammation, PPIs can improve your health. But the indiscriminate overprescribing of them—research suggests the drugs are unnecessary in as many as 80 percent of people taking them—actually causes chronic health problems and increases the overall prevalence of viral infections in the population. An acid blocker may seem like a great idea if you have reflux, especially because it takes the brakes off of what and when you can eat. That newfound freedom of being able to partake in previously problematic foods can be really appealing. But just because something works doesn't mean it's a good idea. Suppressing your body's feedback is almost always a double-edged sword, allowing you to indulge more freely but at a price. In the case of PPIs, the price may be pneumonia, COVID, the flu, or spending your cruise-ship vacation vomiting below deck instead of lounging above.

PPIs and Viruses

In 2020, a large national health survey involving over 53,000 patients found that once daily use of PPIs was associated with double the risk of testing positive for COVID, and almost quadruple the risk in people taking it twice daily. Not only are you much more likely to test positive, but if you're on a PPI and infected with SARS-CoV-2, you're also much more likely to have a severe outcome. Another study with over 100,000 participants reported that PPIs were associated with a 79 percent greater risk of severe clinical outcomes in hospitalized COVID patients, including acute respiratory distress syndrome.

But it's not just COVID that's a concern; blocking stomach acid also increases the chances you'll come down with rotavirus, influenza virus, norovirus, and Middle East respiratory coronavirus infections, and puts you at high risk for contracting acute viral gastroenteritis. Unfortunately, even physicians and sophisticated consumers often don't connect the dots between these common medications that are so frequently prescribed and the increased likelihood of viral infection.

Now that you're clear on the importance of stomach acid for fighting viruses and how acid-blocking drugs can make you more susceptible to them, let's take a look at another frequently overlooked weapon in your anti-viral gut arsenal. Here's a hint: in addition to protecting you from viruses, this next defense system is actually what allows your stomach to be able to excrete large amounts of acid without any damage to the stomach lining itself.

MUCUS

If you live in a cold climate, you're used to having a runny nose in the winter. Cold, dry air irritates your nasal lining, and as a result, the glands in your nose produce extra mucus to keep things moist. Mucus is mostly water, with a little bit of salt and polymers, described by cystic fibrosis researcher Richard C. Boucher as "a cross between Jell-O and glue." It lines surfaces like your eyes, nose, mouth, throat, lungs, and intestines, which are in contact with the outside world, keeping them moist and healthy. But mucus plays a much bigger starring role than just a lubricant; one of its most important functions is to protect you from infections. Microscopic bristles in mucus ensnare viruses in its sticky matrix, which then get coughed or snorted out, or swallowed and inactivated by stomach acid. Like prey imprisoned in a spiderweb, pathogens find it hard to evade mucus's extensive network—unless they have a helping hand.

Although you may associate mucus with the respiratory tract, it's actually your digestive tract, not your lungs, where most of your body's 1.5 liters a day of mucus is made by specialized cells in the lining of your gut called goblet cells. In both the gut and the lungs, viruses have to penetrate this overlying mucus layer to gain access to the cells they're trying to infect below. The protective barrier that mucus provides is five thousand times the diameter of a poliovirus particle. The analogy would be a human wading through 150 gel-filled football fields to reach the end zone and score a touchdown.

Mucus is like your body's own flypaper. It lines the internal surfaces of your body, including your nose, upper and lower respiratory system, and gut, trapping irritants and germs. But mucus doesn't just trap stuff, it's also loaded with protective proteins that can kill and disable viruses. Once trapped, viruses are removed by hairlike projections on cells in the lungs, called cilia, that beat in rhythmic waves to move pathogens up and out of the body. Coughing and sneezing help with the expulsion, and so does stomach acid, since much of the mucus ends up being swallowed.

My patient Claire is very familiar with what happens when mucus doesn't function properly. She has an inherited disorder that affects the cells that produce mucus, sweat, and digestive juices—all fluids that are normally pretty thin and slippery. In people like Claire with cystic fibrosis (CF), a defective gene causes their secretions to become super thick. Normal mucus is about 98 percent water, but Claire's is only 79 percent. Her thick immobile mucus makes it hard for her to breathe, and also harder for her to cough up pathogens, which makes her super susceptible to viral (and bacterial) infections.

You may never have considered that the drippy, runny nose you find so bothersome is actually keeping you safe from viruses. But there are some additional variables in mucus—besides how thick it is—that can affect viral transmission, and those factors impact not only who gets a virus, but also who gives it.

The Role of Mucus in Spreading

On March 10, 2020, sixty-one members of the Skagit Valley Chorale gathered for their evening practice at Mount Vernon Presbyterian Church in Washington State. The governor's order banning large gatherings and requiring everyone to stay home due to the rising cases of COVID was still two weeks away, and mask-wearing wasn't yet on the radar. The conscientious members of the choir took some precautions (no hugging or handshakes), but they were together for two and a half hours in close proximity, they shared snacks, and they spent most of their time singing—a high-risk activity that can transmit viruses in aerosolized mucus and mouth secretions. Days before, on March 7, one member of the group noticed flu-like symptoms.

One person infected with the original SARS-CoV-2 virus would typically infect two to three other people at a gathering. Of the sixty choir members, fifty-three developed COVID, an astoundingly high transmission rate of 88 percent. Even among close contact family members living under the same roof, in the early days of the virus transmission rates were usually only about 20 percent.

You probably remember reading about other high-profile superspreader events—they may seem rare, but historically they're the main drivers of transmission in viral outbreaks—including the recent COVID pandemic, where the initial vast majority of cases were linked to a relatively small portion of infected individuals. In the most recent Ebola outbreak, 3 percent of infected patients accounted for more than 60 percent of all infections, and with measles outbreaks, we know one super-spreader can infect upward of twenty people in a single day.

Super-spreader events aren't explained by any viral mutations, and they aren't predictable based on viral behavior. You can have a huge gathering where very few people, if any, contract the virus, or a small family event where everyone gets it. Close contact and being indoors tell part of the story, and talking a lot or singing definitely doesn't help, but none of those factors explains why when some people sneeze on you, they transmit a virus, and when others overshare their respiratory secretions, nothing happens. Turns out this is less about the virus and more about the mucus of the person doing the sharing. Differences in the composition of the proteins that make up mucus, known as mucins, can dramatically influence the spread of viruses.

In addition to the physical ability to trap viral invaders, mucus also contains enzymes that can degrade viral proteins and antibodies that can neutralize them. Mucins in both saliva and breast milk have anti-viral activity that can inhibit even potent viruses like HIV. If you get sneezed on by someone who was exposed to a virus, but whose mucus has potent anti-viral activity, you're much less likely to get infected. And the converse is also true: super-spreaders likely have mucus that's less toxic to viruses, and that's why they're so good at spreading them around.

Just as some people are really good at spreading viruses, some people are really good at receiving them. The structure and composition of mucus can also predict "super recipients" who are at higher risk of becoming infected when exposed to a virus. Different patterns on mucins may restrict or enhance the binding of a virus to its receptor on the epithelial cells below, so your mucin "signature" may correlate with a positive or a negative outcome from viral infection.

Depending on the physical and chemical characteristics of your mucus, you may be a super-spreader, a super recipient, or super immune to ever becoming infected if you have the super good kind of anti-viral mucus.

Internal factors like your genetics and immune system influence the composition of your mucins, but external environmental factors and lifestyle play a role, too. So here again are several host factors involved in viral infectivity that you can control to mitigate your risk. By cultivating healthy mucus through not smoking, getting plenty of exposure to clean air, eating a healthy diet, and drinking lots of water, you can decrease your chances of symptomatic infection. It may not sound important, high-tech, or cutting-edge, but having good-quality effective mucus that can trap and expel viruses is another one of your critical host defenses.

PROTECTING YOU AND YOUR PROGENY

One area where mucin research is already extraordinarily helpful is in obstetrics. When mucin's structure changes, its ability to fight pathogens can become compromised. This can be due to differences in the chemical properties of the mucins or the actual physical strength of the mucus itself. An example where we routinely use mucus as a diagnostic tool is to assess the risk of preterm birth. If you're pregnant and your cervical mucus is thinner and more permeable than normal, it can allow more pathogens to penetrate through, travel up to your uterus, and infect your fetus, putting you at higher risk of preterm birth. Thicker mucus, on the other hand, indicates a lower risk of preterm birth. Just by doing a simple vaginal exam and feeling the cervical mucus with their fingers, doctors can accurately predict whether a woman is at risk for preterm birth and needs to be monitored more closely. In these circumstances quality mucus doesn't just protect the mom from viruses—it helps keep her unborn child safe, too.

Let It Flow

If you've ever had trouble sleeping at night because you're hacking up a bunch of mucus, you've probably considered reaching for a cough suppressant. In the late 1800s, the pharmaceutical company Bayer started promoting a new cough formula as a better and safer alternative to previous options, despite the fact that it contained heroin. Mrs. Winslow's Soothing Syrup had been launched in Maine in 1849 with ingredients like sodium carbonate and water—plus a whopping dose of morphine. It transformed irritable crying children into peaceful sleepers, but tragically, some of them never woke up. Cough syrups these days contain pretty benign ingredients compared to a century ago, but they can still be a danger to your health. Cough suppressants can actually make you sicker because they diminish your ability to cough up viruses and other pathogens and expel them from your body. Suppressing your cough reflex can end up turning a minor problem in your upper airway into a more severe one deep in your lungs. The American Academy of Pediatrics recommends: "cough and cold medicines should not be prescribed, recommended or used for respiratory illnesses in young children." That's good advice for adults and older children, too. As annoying as it is to lie next to someone who's hacking away in bed, remember that their cough is protecting them, even as they sleep—and keep you awake!

Mucus and the coughing that helps expel it are an important route for your body to eliminate viruses, and now you know that interfering with that process can leave you more vulnerable to getting sick. Like a hacking cough or a runny nose, this next defense mechanism is one that many people mistakenly think of as a dangerous symptom that needs to be extinguished, rather than an effective means for your body to do battle with viral interlopers.

HEAT

A fever is a temporary increase in your body temperature above 100.4°F.

It happens when your body's internal thermostat—found in a part of your brain called the hypothalamus—raises the temperature above its normal level, usually in response to an infection or illness. Although you may think of a fever as a sign that you're ill (and you'd usually be right), fever is also a sure sign that your body is working overtime to protect you.

Our perception of fever has changed a lot over the centuries and continues to evolve. Early civilizations thought fever was induced by devilish spirits, and sometimes used exorcism to rid the body of "evil humors" to try to return temperatures to normal and cleanse the soul. Most ancient physicians took a different view, seeing fever as more helpful than harmful. Fever therapy dates back to thousands of years ago and includes Hippocrates among its fans, who famously said, "Give me a fever, and I can cure any disease," after noting the calming effects of malarial fever in epileptics. In 1927, the Austrian neuropsychiatrist Julius Wagner-Jauregg received the Nobel Prize in Medicine for his work using fever therapy to treat dementia in neurosyphilis, a practice that was in use until the 1950s. Fever therapy is still used today in many cultures in the form of saunas, sweat lodges, and steam baths.

To Treat or Not to Treat?

Fever is both a signal from your body to alert you that it's fighting something and a part of its protective mechanism, and the question we should be asking isn't whether to feed or starve it, but whether we should be treating it at all. In the 1800s, the science of microbiology and the realization that fever could be a sign of infection, coupled with the discovery that animals could die quickly when their body temperature exceeded a certain level, created an association among fever, disease, and death. It also helped pave the way for the widespread use of fever-lowering drugs known as antipyretics. These days we tend to instinctively treat a fever, especially in children, because of a perception that it's harmful and may lead to complications, without ever considering that the opposite might be true: that in fact fever might be an important health-preserving host defense and interfering with it may leave you more rather than less vulnerable to viral infection.

FEVER AND CHILDREN

If you've ever taken care of a screaming child with a temperature of 102°F, you know it can be a traumatic experience. There are two primary reasons why doctors and anxious parents treat a fever: to reduce the risk of febrile seizures, and to relieve discomfort. In a very small percentage of children, a high temperature can cause brief benign seizures that typically occur on the first day of the fever, last a few minutes, are usually harmless, and don't cause brain damage or death. But despite the fact that they're often recommended by pediatricians, antipyretics aren't effective at preventing febrile seizures. Like antibiotics given to children with viral infections, they're often being prescribed to calm worried parents who expect a remedy, not because they're medically indicated. The discomfort that we often attribute to a fever is almost always due to the illness behind the fever, and too much focus on bringing down a high temperature can detract from the real work of finding and treating the underlying cause.

More Good Than Harm

Fever has been conserved over thousands of years of evolution as a response to infection, which is strong evidence that it provides an advantage for the host. Let's take a closer look at what those advantages may be.

Most viruses stop replicating at high temperatures, so fever is an incredibly important way for your body to prevent further attack and damage. Here's just how important: the replication rate of poliovirus at normal body temperatures is 250 times higher than at an elevated temperature of 104°F—a clear example of your host defenses working to stop the spread of the virus within your body. In addition to stopping viral replication in its tracks, fever increases the mobilization of your immune cells, which release virus-fighting antibodies and send out help signals to other inflammatory cells to come join the battle. Like a heat-seeking missile finding its target, fever enhances the ability of white blood cells to destroy pathogens. The reality is that when you're battling a virus and reach for a pharmaceutical agent to lower your temperature, you're actually sabotaging one of your most important— and most potent—anti-viral weapons.

It's important to remember that fever is a physiologic response, not an illness. It can also be an important signal that there's something we need to pay attention to—like COVID, where fever is often the only sign of infection early on, and one you could easily miss if you were taking antipyretics like aspirin, acetaminophen, or NSAIDs (nonsteroidal anti-inflammatory drugs). Viral infections are often associated with a low-grade fever, but some, like dengue, can cause high fevers, too. There's no way to know based on temperature alone whether you're dealing with a viral or bacterial infection, but in both cases, a fever is part of your body's attempt to kill the invading organism, and using medication to suppress it can actually make things worse. Antipyretics like ibuprofen and acetaminophen have been associated with prolonged influenza infection, they can worsen symptoms during the common cold, and in some studies they've been found to delay the resolution of chickenpox. We're often anxiously watching the mercury rise (or the digits increase) on the thermometer when we should probably be worried about it dipping below normal. In children with viral meningitis, a low temperature (hypothermia) is strongly associated with dying, while a high fever is associated with better outcomes, again validating what we know about the ability of elevated body temperature to slow down or halt viral replication.

It's worth emphasizing again that fever isn't caused by viruses—it's caused by your body's response to them, and that response is designed to fight and kill pathogens. Like muscle aches, hangovers, and heartburn, fever has been positively selected by evolution because for most of us, the benefits far outweigh the risks. Of course there are times and clinical scenarios when fever can be harmful, but research over the last several decades suggests an overall protective role that includes blocking viral replication, enhancing your immune system to respond more effectively to a viral threat, and, as you'll learn in the next section, even creating physical changes in your gut that deter viruses.

Beyond the potential benefit to the individual of letting a fever run its course, suppressing fever in normal clinical settings may lead to negative effects for society as a whole, due to a possible increase in the spread of infections when you bring the body temperature back down to normal and thereby allow viral replication to proceed unchecked.

The Gut-Fever Connection

Your gut lining is normally permeable, allowing passage of nutrients in and cellular waste matter out. In the face of viral attack, fever communicates to the cells lining your gut that it's time to tighten up in order to create a more impenetrable barrier that can resist invasion. The gut lining becomes temporarily less permeable in the setting of a fever, which has the benefit of making it harder for viruses to pass through. Suppressing that communication with an antipyretic can lead to a more permeable gut lining and increased susceptibility to viral attack.

Your gut microbiome also responds to changes in core temperature. Housing laboratory mice at cool temperatures leads to changes in their microbiome that help them stay warm, but those changes also divert resources away from fighting infection. The increased core temperature that fever provides means mice (and humans) don't have to worry about trying to raise their body temperature to warm up and can get on with the business of battling pathogens. We don't know the specific microbial changes in humans that occur in response to a fever, but research suggests that those changes are synergistic with enhanced responses in your immune system that fever elicits—all with the same goal of protecting you.

Thermal Therapy

In addition to killing viruses, it turns out that fever is pretty good at getting rid of cancer cells, too—something old that's new again revamped as "thermal therapy." Like viruses, cancer cells are more susceptible to high heat than normal cells. Fever can inhibit the growth of certain tumors by damaging the metabolism of those cancer cells and also enhance cancer-dissolving enzymes and immune cells, which have increased activity at high temperatures. There have even been reports of Hodgkin's lymphoma going into remission after fever from viral infections like measles.

With age, our ability to develop fever decreases and so does the strength of our immune system, making the elderly particularly vulnerable to infections. Death from COVID is usually a result of acute respiratory distress syndrome (ARDS), which kills off lung cells. In an experimental ARDS rat model, several hours of fever stopped cell death and protected lung cells from the inflammatory damage of SARS-CoV-2. In the right setting, thermal therapy may be a way to protect vulnerable populations like the elderly from the complications of viral infections, essentially creating a protective fever for them when their body can't do it on its own.

WHEN THINGS GO WRONG

Our bodies have an amazing capacity to wage war on viruses: we can inactivate them with acid, we can trap and expel them in mucus, and we can halt their replication with a fever. These are incredibly well-designed systems that, when allowed to function properly without interference, can keep you safe in the face of harmful viral exposure. When you add in the powerful virus-fighting capacity of your army of gut bacteria, plus the battalions of immune cells they're able to muster, it truly is an impressive array of anti-viral capabilities.

But what happens when there is interference, intentional or inadvertent, and instead of having a strong gut shield, you find yourself defenseless and vulnerable to viral attack? The first order of business is making sure you're familiar with how and why things went awry, and the second is knowing how to get them back on track. In the next section, we're going to be covering just that.

To view the scientific references cited in this chapter, please visit

drrobynnechutkan.com/anti-viral-gut-references.

WHAT GOES WRONG

PART 2

4

Good Guts Gone Bad: Understanding Dysbiosis

Every day we live and every meal we eat we influence the great microbial organ inside us—for better or for worse.

—Giulia Enders, *Gut: The Inside Story of Our Body's Most Underrated Organ*

If I asked you what the number one risk factor for getting COVID and having a poor outcome is, you'd probably say heart disease or a chronic lung condition, or being elderly or obese or diabetic, or maybe having cancer or taking a medication that suppresses your immune system. And you'd be correct that those are all conditions and situations that make you more susceptible and can definitely lead to worse outcomes. But by far the most accurate predictor of whether you survive unscathed, have lasting symptoms, or die during a viral pandemic is in your gut. In order to understand why, let's take a closer look at a disease state that millions of us suffer from without even knowing it.

DYSBIOSIS

The name sounds a bit dystopian, but the definition of dysbiosis is pretty simple: it's a microbial imbalance in your gut where you have overgrowth of harmful species and underrepresentation of helpful ones. While there's incredible microbial variation from person to person, our health depends on having an appropriate balance, without any one species becoming unnaturally dominant or submissive, and with essential bacteria present in sufficient numbers. If you want to be able to resist pathogens, then you must nurture and preserve your ultimate fighting machine: a rich and diverse microbiome.

How exactly does dysbiosis make you more vulnerable to viral infection? Your microbiome regulates your host defense responses and your immunity, which determine your outcome when infected by a virus. These interactions affect viral replication, transmission, and severity of infection, and they're all influenced by the composition and diversity of your gut flora. Your microbiome has all sorts of ways it can lessen illness after a viral infection, by both enhancing your immunity and reducing the virus's replication and infectivity.

Here are a couple of real-life examples: *Staphylococcus epidermidis,* a common bacteria found in your nose, can suppress replication of influenza A virus (IAV) in your nasal mucosa, which prevents spread to your lungs. *Staphylococcus aureus,* which commonly colonizes your upper respiratory tract, also helps protect you by significantly decreasing IAV-mediated lung injury. If you've been taking frequent antibiotics, chances are the antibiotics will have wiped out these two bacteria and you'll be more likely to develop serious lung complications like pneumonia from influenza. Another example of your microbiome looking out for you occurs with norovirus infection, the most common cause of acute gastroenteritis. People infected with norovirus usually develop vomiting, diarrhea, and stomach cramping, but if your microbiome is rich in helpful *Bacteroidetes* species and low in pathogenic *Clostridia,* you're much more likely to be asymptomatic if you encounter norovirus. Women with high levels of protective *Lactobacillus* species in their vagina are at much lower risk of becoming infected after exposure to HIV, HPV, and other STDs because the bacteria produce acid that repels the viruses. Having a lot of

Faecalibacterium prausnitzii in your microbiome is associated with a much better prognosis from COVID, in part because the bacteria actually drives the SARS-CoV-2 virus toward reduced virulence. These are some of the many ways the composition of your microbiome can affect your outcome when you encounter a virus.

To treat or prevent viral infections, we mainly rely on two interventions: anti-viral drugs and vaccines, and there's evidence that your microbiome can affect the response to both. For example, dysbiosis in the vaginal microbiome reduces the efficacy of some anti-viral drugs against HIV. Within a population, vaccines show enormous variations in their efficacy, and one of the variables that controls that efficacy is differences in the microbiome among individuals. In infants, *Actinobacteria* species increase the response to hepatitis B virus vaccines, while a less healthy microbial profile that includes large amounts of *Enterobacteria, Pseudomonas,* and *Clostridia* species decreases it. What all these examples illustrate is that it's not bad luck that leads to wins or losses in the battle against viruses—it's predictable (and usually preventable) changes in your microbiome.

DETECTING DYSBIOSIS

Now that you know that dysbiosis is such a major risk factor for viral illness and complications, I want you to get familiar with its signs and symptoms. The manifestations of dysbiosis can be far-reaching and varied: fatigue, difficulty losing (or gaining) weight, food intolerances and cravings, bloating, constipation, diarrhea, yeast overgrowth, vaginal discharge, acne, rosacea, rashes, mood disorders, and lots of other symptoms have their origins in dysbiosis. It may also be the root cause or a contributing factor behind many poorly understood and difficult to diagnose medical conditions, including some autoimmune diseases, leaky gut, irritable bowel syndrome (IBS), small intestinal bacterial overgrowth (SIBO), and myalgic encephalomyelitis/chronic fatigue syndrome (ME/CFS), which has so much in common with post-viral syndromes like long COVID. A shared feature of all these conditions is bacterial imbalance. (For a detailed and comprehensive overview of the medical conditions and manifestations of dysbiosis, check out my second book, *The Microbiome Solution*.)

DYSBIOSIS MAY BE THE ROOT CAUSE BEHIND
- Autoimmune diseases
- Bloating
- Celiac/gluten sensitivity
- Chronic fatigue syndrome
- Depression
- Food allergies and sensitivities
- Food cravings
- Inflammatory bowel disease (IBD)
- Irritable bowel syndrome (IBS)
- Leaky gut
- Parasites
- Post-viral syndromes
- Skin conditions (acne, rosacea, eczema)
- Small intestinal bacterial overgrowth (SIBO)
- Vaginosis
- Weight gain
- Yeast overgrowth

Dysbiosis can be a challenging diagnosis to make because although there are a few tests that may provide supporting evidence, it's primarily a clinical diagnosis that's based on careful history taking and familiarity with the wide spectrum of symptoms it can cause. Because you can't see it or test for it the way you can with conditions like gallstones or colon cancer, and because it's largely a result of our own overzealous medical practices, mainstream medicine is only now beginning to recognize dysbiosis as a real condition, despite the fact that millions of people suffer from it. Getting thrush in your mouth or a vaginal yeast infection after a round of antibiotics is a classic example of dysbiosis—your native yeast population proliferates unchecked to fill the void created by the disappearance of large numbers of essential bacteria.

Millions of Americans suffer from dysbiosis because the factors that damage our gut bacteria are so widespread. Antibiotics aren't the only threat; our highly processed and pesticized food chain puts our microbes at risk, and so does our daily diet filled with too much fat, too little fiber, too much alcohol, and sugary drinks that feed the wrong microbes. Not to mention edible substances we consume all the time without realizing their detrimental effects, like artificial sweeteners that can turn normal helpful bacteria into pathogens. Plus, microbe-depleting medications, acid blockers that disrupt the pH of the gut, our toxin-filled environment, and our sedentary, stressful, overscheduled lives can all be major microbial disrupters. Let's take a closer look at how some of these everyday practices can create dysbiosis and make us more vulnerable to viruses.

COMMON CAUSES OF DYSBIOSIS
Medications
You may think of your medicine cabinet as the place to go for solutions to what ails you, but when it comes to dysbiosis, it's often the source of the problem. A major review published in the journal *Nature* in 2020 analyzed forty-one different categories of medication and found that nineteen were associated with significant disturbances in the microbiome. In addition to disrupting your gut flora, some of

these medications have other side effects that make you more vulnerable to viruses. Here are some of the top offenders:

Antibiotics prevent death from serious bacterial infection every day, but in our current climate of overdiagnosis and overtreatment, they're also tremendously overutilized or misused in a few ways: for minor self-limited infections that will resolve on their own, as a preventative measure for infections that are unlikely to ever occur, and for viral infections against which they're completely ineffective. Conservative estimates from the CDC suggest that as much as half of all antibiotic use is inappropriate, leading to unnecessary side effects, higher costs, and bacterial "superbugs" resistant to every known antibiotic that threaten to plunge us back into the dark ages of medicine. But as we've just learned, overzealous antibiotic use also creates another serious problem—it dramatically increases your chances of viral infection and worsens your prognosis if you do get infected by removing critical species that are intimately involved in your anti-viral response. The startling statistic is that just five days of a broad-spectrum antibiotic like the kind used to treat a sinus or urinary tract infection can remove up to one-third of your gut bacteria. That includes whatever bacterial pathogen you're trying to kill, plus droves of helpful species that play an important role in your ability to fight viruses. When you destroy these essential microbes, you allow more pathogenic ones that are normally present in low amounts to flourish, and the result is dysbiosis.

The reality is that most of us with a healthy gut can tolerate a course of antibiotics every couple of years, but we may have a difficult time recovering from more frequent use. For those who receive more than two rounds of broad-spectrum antibiotics a year or who take longer courses, or whose microbiome is still forming (young children), the drugs can do serious and sometimes lasting damage to the immune system. In my practice, I see major problems with recurrent viral infections in people who've been treated with months (and sometimes years!) of antibiotics for problems like chronic Lyme disease, recurrent sinusitis, or acne. And for those of us who've fed our microbes a steady diet of low-fiber processed food, our ability to bounce back from antibiotics is even more limited. In the second part of this book, I'll provide you with a list of critical questions to ask your doctor before taking an antibiotic, plus steps to help reduce their side effects when avoidance just isn't possible.

Proton pump inhibitors (PPIs) like Nexium, Prilosec, Prevacid, AcipHex, and Protonix are really good at what they do: getting rid of stomach acid. That might bring relief if you have acid reflux, but it comes at a price. As we discussed in the previous chapter, normally the acid in your stomach inhibits bacterial growth, keeping numbers much lower in your upper gastrointestinal (GI) tract compared to down in your colon. That natural gradient of increasing amounts of gut bacteria as you travel from the top (stomach) to the bottom (colon) of the gut is important for normal microbiome function, and disrupting it with long-term use of PPIs (more than eight weeks at a time) is a major cause of dysbiosis. Not to mention losing the anti-viral effects of stomach acid that normally inactivates viral DNA.

Nonsteroidal anti-inflammatory drugs (NSAIDs) like Motrin, Advil, and Aleve are among the most commonly prescribed drugs in the world for a reason—they help relieve fever, pain, and inflammation. But like many other "wonder drugs," that relief comes at the expense of your gut. While

NSAIDs don't have direct antimicrobial activity, by changing the chemical environment in your gut and causing erosions and ulceration, they interfere with microbial metabolism and can precipitate dysbiosis.

Birth control pills are the most common form of contraception in the United States today and are used by millions of women for reasons besides preventing pregnancy, such as to decrease menstrual cramps, clear up acne, treat endometriosis, and reduce symptoms of premenstrual syndrome. Unfortunately, both birth control pills and **hormone replacement therapy** increase estrogen levels, which affect your microbial ecosystem and can lead to chronic yeast infections and other signs of dysbiosis.

Corticosteroids, like prednisone, are used to treat almost every form of inflammation. They don't cure most conditions but can suppress symptoms, making them hugely popular, especially for hard-to-treat autoimmune disorders where there often aren't many pharmaceutical options. Steroids are a major cause of dysbiosis because they suppress friendly bacteria and allow the proliferation of fungal species, which increases your susceptibility to viral infections. Oral or intravenous forms of steroids are more detrimental to the microbiome than topical forms, but long-term use of inhaled steroids or steroid creams and ointments can also affect your microbiome and leave you vulnerable to viral infections.

Chemotherapy should ideally just kill cancer cells and leave the rest of your body alone. Unfortunately, when these powerful drugs do their job of poisoning cells, lots of microbes are affected, too. That may help explain why secondary cancers are so common after chemotherapy and why people have such a hard time regaining their health after treatment. In addition to weakening the immune system, certain forms of chemo can also cause lung problems like fibrosis and inflammation, which could worsen your prognosis if you get a respiratory viral infection.

Diet

My definition of food is very simple: something that nourishes you. That means it should nourish your gut bacteria, too, since a thriving microbiome is the key to good health. In addition to needing specific raw materials and nutrients in order to survive, gut bacteria also need to be protected from toxins and chemicals in food, and from the wrong types of food that can create imbalance. The Anti-Viral Gut Plan tells you exactly what to add to your diet, what to remove, and what to replace it with, to make sure you're feeding your microbes exactly what they need. Here's an overview of some of the problematic foods that can wreak havoc in your microbiome that you should go out of your way to avoid:

Artificial sweeteners claim to save you calories because they aren't absorbed in your small intestine, but they still cause the release of insulin—a hormone that tells your cells to store calories as fat—and some even have carcinogenic effects. But unexpected weight gain and cancer aren't their only drawbacks. Artificial sweeteners are fermented in the colon, a process that, in addition to producing lots of bloat-causing gas, also damages your gut bacteria. Research published in the *International Journal of Molecular Sciences* in 2021 showed that in addition to their previously known deleterious effects on the number and type of bacteria in your gut, several common artificial sweeteners like saccharin, sucralose, and aspartame can cause healthy gut bacteria to become diseased and invade the gut wall, potentially leading to serious health issues like inflammation and food allergies.

Sugar and fat are major microbial disrupters. A sugary, starchy, fat-laden diet can send bad bacteria into a feeding frenzy and encourage growth of the wrong type of bacteria in your gut. That can lead to dysbiosis and lay the foundation for lots of different diseases, including worse outcomes from viral illnesses. We'll explore the profound differences in the microbiome produced by a high-fat/high-sugar diet versus a high-fiber one later in the chapter.

Alcohol is tricky. We can argue about whether a glass or two of red wine may be good for your heart, but don't try to convince yourself it's helping your microbiome—or your ability to fight infection. Studies show that just one drink per day in women and two in men can induce dysbiosis, damage your liver, increase permeability of your gut, and affect your immune system. When you're exposed to a virus, your body mounts an immune response to attack and kill it. In general, the healthier your immune system, the quicker it can clear the virus and the faster you can recover. Alcohol makes it harder for your immune system to do its job defending you against pathogens. In the lungs, alcohol damages immune cells that are responsible for clearing the virus out of your airway. In the gut, it triggers inflammation and destroys microorganisms that maintain immune health, leading to an increased risk of infections and complications. If you're at high risk for viral infections (older, immunocompromised, obese, have autoimmune disease or diabetes) or trying to recover from post-viral symptoms, abstinence is definitely the way to go.

Frankenfood is a not particularly complimentary term for genetically modified foods, reflecting the concern many in the medical field have about their health effects. Genetic modification takes the genetic material from one organism and inserts it into the permanent genetic code of another, creating novel substances such as potatoes with bacteria genes, pigs with human genes, and fish with cattle genes. This process has been used to alter many food items, including much of our corn, soy, and sugar, and canola and cottonseed oils. Several studies indicate that eating foods that are genetically modified to tolerate the use of herbicides like glyphosate cause problematic changes in our gut bacteria. Glyphosate causes dysbiosis in poultry, which in turn increases the incidence of pathogens like *Salmonella* in the animals, and it's also associated with dysbiosis in cows that are fed genetically modified corn. Since more than 70 percent of processed foods on supermarket shelves today contain genetically engineered ingredients, it's likely that these foods are having a similar effect on our microbiome.

This long list I just provided might seem theoretical, but the reality is that thousands, if not millions, of people succumb unnecessarily to viral illnesses because they regularly ingest foods and medications that are harmful to their microbiome.

. . . . .

Whether you've already been diagnosed with dysbiosis or one of its associated conditions or are still trying to figure out the cause of unexplained symptoms, here's a checklist of questions that can help you identify whether something may have gone wrong with your microbiome. Answering yes to even one of these questions could indicate you have dysbiosis, and the risk is cumulative based on how many risk factors you have.

DYSBIOSIS CHECKLIST

❑ Have you taken broad-spectrum antibiotics more than four times per year or for longer than two weeks at a time?

❑ Do you take corticosteroids such as prednisone at a dose of more than 20 milligrams per day?

❑ Are you on acid suppressive therapy with proton pump inhibitors?

❑ Do you take birth control pills or hormone replacement therapy?

❑ Have you been on chemotherapy in the last five years?

❑ Do you take ibuprofen, aspirin, or other NSAIDs regularly?

❑ Are you a picky eater who rarely eats green vegetables?

❑ Do you follow a low-carbohydrate diet that restricts grains, legumes, or fruit?

❑ Do you consume large amounts of sugar and starchy foods?

❑ Do you drink more than ten alcoholic beverages per week?

❑ Do you drink one or more sodas or diet sodas daily?

❑ Do you regularly eat food that's been treated with pesticides like glyphosate?

❑ Do you use products like antibacterial soaps and body washes, or deodorants, mouthwashes, and toothpastes that contain the microbe-disrupting chemical triclosan?

These risk factors and the damage they can do to your microbiome aren't obvious from the outside. You would never have looked at my patient Alicia and guessed that she is someone who would have a poor outcome from a viral illness like COVID, but her microbiome told a different story.

Before I met her, Alicia had taken over thirty courses of antibiotics for sinus infections, and that eventually led to frequent vaginal yeast infections. A naturopathic doctor prescribed eight weeks of a potent antifungal called fluconazole, which helped clear up her vaginal discharge but didn't improve her bloating, gas, or constipation. The naturopath also put her on a strict diet that excluded all grains, fruit, starchy vegetables, sugar, honey, and sweeteners of any kind, and she had been eating only meat, chicken, eggs, and a few green vegetables for the last two years.

I tried to reassure Alicia that her GI symptoms were more likely the result of her restricted low-fiber diet, plus insufficient quantities of essential bacteria as a result of all of the antibiotics, rather than due to yeast overgrowth, but she was fervent in her belief that yeast was the problem and needed additional treatment. Persuading Alicia to stop the fluconazole was a lot easier than getting her to liberalize her diet. She and her gut bacteria desperately needed some fiber, but she was petrified of eating carbohydrates, even high-fiber complex carbs. She'd read that carbs feed yeast species and wasn't aware that indigestible plant fiber is actually critical for cultivating healthy gut microbes that keep yeast species under control.

Alicia was one of my first patients to get COVID, and because she was young (forty-three), slim, a nonsmoker, and had no history of heart disease, high blood pressure, or diabetes, she initially wasn't too worried. I have to admit, I was surprised when her husband called to tell me she'd been admitted to the ICU, and even more shocked when I learned she had succumbed to the virus after being in the hospital for three weeks. The medical team taking care of her had suspected (but not proven) bacterial pneumonia superinfection and had blasted her with antibiotics and eventually high doses of steroids when she didn't respond. In retrospect, it's likely that Alicia's underlying depletion of gut bacteria due to previous antibiotic use plus her low-fiber diet had made her more susceptible to getting COVID in the first place, and the subsequent heavy-duty antibiotics combined with steroids in the hospital compromised her immune system further. The tragic end result was a gut shield that was so damaged that it was unable to protect her from the virus.

YOUR GUT SHIELD

I tell you this story not to scare you but to emphasize that it's not your outward appearance that's important when it comes to viral infections; it's what's going on inside your gut with the health of your microbiome, and that's not always evident externally. Simply put, a healthier gut microbiome means a more benign course of viral illness—or none at all. It also means a lower risk of microbial abnormalities persisting after the virus is gone that play a role in the prolonged symptoms many people experience after viral illnesses like hepatitis, mono, and COVID. Dysbiosis is the foundation on which viral susceptibility is built, and avoiding or remediating it is the key to creating a healthy anti-viral gut.

But how do you actually achieve optimal microbial health? What do you need to do to strengthen that invisible but essential gut shield inside your body in order to stave off viruses? The good news, and what makes me so optimistic about the work that I do, is that your microbiome is constantly changing, and improvements in the composition of your gut bacteria can have a profound impact on your health and ability to resist infection. The bacteria you start the week with on a Monday morning can be totally different from the ones you've cultivated by Friday afternoon. Those improvements in your microbial richness and diversity also impact what genes in your body get turned on and off, which can influence disease expression and can have huge implications for outcomes after viral infections. So how exactly should you be caring for your microbes so that they can take care of you? In the previous section I pointed out some foods—and edible food-like substances—that can cause problems in your microbiome. Now let's take a look at what you *should* be eating if you're trying to cultivate an anti-viral gut.

A Tale of Two Cities

The local diet in Boulpon, Burkina Faso, a rural hamlet in the western part of Africa, hasn't changed much in the last ten thousand years. Villagers from the Mossi ethnic group still practice subsistence farming like their Neolithic ancestors did. Their main meal is a thick porridge made from millet and sorghum that they grind into a pulp on a flat stone and eat with vegetables and herbs. Overall, their diet is high in fiber, with very little animal protein or fat. Staples include grains, cereals, legumes like black-eyed peas, and vegetables. In the rainy season, termites make an occasional appearance on the menu, and on special occasions, one of the chickens that roam around the village ends up in someone's pot.

On the other side of the world, the Mediterranean diet has been celebrated as one of the healthiest ways to eat, with lots of fruits, vegetables, legumes, nuts, seeds, lean protein like fish, healthy fats like olive oil, and minimal red meat and sugar. It's how people in Spain, Italy, and Greece ate for centuries and explains why they had lower rates of heart disease and were overall healthier compared to their peers in northern Europe and the United States. Nowadays, modern Italians eat very differently from their ancestors. In cities like Florence, they have largely adopted a Western diet with lots of meat and dairy, plus large amounts of processed carbohydrates like bread, pasta, and sugar that are low in fiber.

Dr. Paolo Lionetti, a pediatric gastroenterologist and microbiome researcher at the University of Florence, set out to investigate how the diets in Boulpon and modern-day Florence might affect gut bacteria. His landmark study compared the microbiome in a group of young children from Boulpon and another from Florence to assess the impact of what they ate on the germs growing in their gut.

In Dr. Lionetti's study, all the children were vaginally born, breast-fed, and healthy, so not surprisingly, the microbiome in the two groups was very similar at birth and in infancy. But as soon as the children graduated from breast milk to the local diet, things started to change. The Italian children eating lots of fat and sugar had low microbial diversity—a classic marker for dysbiosis—and they also had an abundance of species associated with allergies, obesity, inflammation, and poor outcomes from viral infections. The African children eating a diet full of high-fiber legumes and vegetables had greater bacterial diversity, more species associated with leanness, and much higher levels of a beneficial by-product of gut bacteria called short-chain fatty acids (SCFAs).

TABLE 4.1 • Short-Chain Fatty Acids

SCFA	MAIN BACTERIAL PRODUCER	HEALTH BENEFITS
Butyrate	• *Faecalibacterium prausnitzii* • *Eubacterium rectale* • *Roseburia*	• Energy source for colon cells • Helps prevent leaky gut • Fights inflammation/cancer • Protects the brain
Propionate	• *Bacteroidetes* • *Firmicutes* • *Lachnospiraceae*	• Regulates appetite • Combats inflammation • Protects against cancer
Acetate	• *Bifidobacteria* • *Lactobacillus* • *Akkermansia*	• Regulates pH of the gut • Controls appetite • Nourishes butyrate-producers • Protects against pathogens
Lactate	• Lactic acid bacteria	• Repels pathogens • Regulates immune system • Fights opportunistic bacteria

SHORT-CHAIN SUPERHEROES

SCFAs are the stars of the show when it comes to a balanced microbiome and good gut health. They're created when certain species of bacteria ferment dietary fibers. In addition to being protective against inflammation, SCFAs play a big role in how bacteria like *Faecalibacterium prausnitzii* help you resist and recover from viruses. In the first chapter I discussed a balanced immune response known as "immune equilibrium." SCFAs orchestrate that equilibrium by suppressing inflammatory responses in your gut and other organs, which helps you successfully recover from viral infections while preventing an overblown immune response.

SCFAs also remotely influence your local immune response to viral infection in your lungs. High levels favor an uneventful recovery, while low levels are associated with complications like asthmatic reactions or bacterial superinfection that can lead to poor outcomes or even death. In mice infected with influenza, high levels of SCFAs increase survival in the infected mice by setting their immune system at a healthy level of responsiveness while blunting harmful excessive immune reactions in their lungs. A Japanese study published in the *American Journal of Rhinology & Allergy* in 2021 found that SCFAs can also reduce the number of virus binding sites in your airways, which may be another way they positively influence your response to viral illnesses like influenza and COVID.

In addition to ensuring a balanced immune response and limiting viral damage in the lungs, SCFAs help maintain the integrity of your gut lining—an important physical barrier to viruses. Low levels of SCFAs increase intestinal permeability, which increases the likelihood of pathogens penetrating through your gut barrier, gaining access to your insides, and making you a lot sicker.

MICROBIAL FOUNDATIONS OF DISEASE

In Dr. Lionetti's study, the children from Burkina Faso had more than double the amount of SCFAs as the Italian children—and much higher levels of the bacteria that produce them. Bacteria like *Faecalibacterium prausnitzii* break down fiber to create SCFAs that serve as an energy source for those same bacteria. It's a synergistic relationship that relies on the consumption of large amounts of plant fiber. The children in Burkina Faso were eating twice as much fiber as the Italian children, and that's why they had such high levels of SCFAs. In the United States, fiber consumption in adults is only 10 to 15 grams daily, about half of the USDA recommendation of 25 grams in women and 38 grams in men. That low fiber intake correlates with low rates of SCFAs, and high rates of diseases like obesity, diabetes, and heart disease. Not enough fiber can be even worse for your microbiome than too much sugar and fat. Certain types of dietary fiber basically feed your microbes and are a crucial part of restoring and maintaining microbial balance. These foods increase the population of helpful species in your gut, while low-fiber diets have the opposite effect.

Despite the dramatic differences in their levels of SCFAs and gut bacteria, none of the children in either group of Dr. Lionetti's study were sick. But the Western diet had already laid the microbial foundations for disease and obesity in the Italian children, while the high-fiber diet of the African children had created a protective microbiome associated with leanness and health that made these diseases much less likely. Childhood obesity rates in Burkina Faso are less than 1 percent. In Italy, the shift away from a traditional way of eating has made people fatter and sicker: one-third of Italian children are overweight or obese (outranking even the United States) and the country has high rates of diabetes, high blood pressure, stroke, and heart disease typical of a "Western" low-fiber diet.

Having a healthier microbiome doesn't mean children in Burkina

Faso are immune to the perils of subsistence farming in a poor country. Malnutrition from not enough food is a major threat, and malaria, tuberculosis, and cholera are among the leading causes of death in that part of the world. But high microbial diversity and lots of SCFAs virtually guarantees them something that the Italian children don't have: protection against the comorbidities that contribute to the death of so many people during viral outbreaks, and an immune system that's primed to handle the threat. It's not drug cocktails and ICU care that are essential in a viral pandemic—it's your own basic host defenses, and those defenses rely on the health of your gut bacteria. They can't protect you if you're feeding them Cheetos.

WHAT TO EAT?

The best diet to eat in order to support an anti-viral gut is one that your good bugs can thrive on. One of the most important of these good bugs is *Faecalibacterium prausnitzii*, a main producer of SCFAs in your gut. In healthy adults, it represents more than 5 percent of your gut microbiome, making it one of the most common gut bacteria. High levels of *F. prausnitzii* are typical of a balanced microbiome—and since high levels also reduce your risk of severe viral illness, *F. prausnitzii* is a species you want to cultivate. You can do this by eating foods like onion, garlic, asparagus, leeks, and others that are high in a type of dietary fiber called inulin. Foods like inulin are what's known as "prebiotics" because they feed your healthy gut bacteria, dramatically increasing your levels of *F. prausnitzii* and SCFAs, and warding off dysbiosis and illness. They are medicinal foods in the true sense, and there's no supplement, over-the-counter medication, prescription drug, or cocktail of high-tech pharmaceuticals that can compare to their regular consumption in safeguarding you against a bad outcome from viral illnesses.

FOODS HIGH IN INULIN

- Artichokes
- Asparagus
- Bananas
- Chicory root
- Dandelion root
- Garlic
- Leeks
- Onions

Food Is Always Best

Store-bought bacteria, butyrate supplements, or even a healthy person's actual microbiome in the form of a transplanted stool sample can't produce the same effect as a high-fiber diet and the natural increase in SCFAs that it generates. And keep in mind that although SCFAs have been determined to be essential to gut health, there are probably dozens, if not hundreds, of other compounds that are likely produced in the process of gut bacteria fermenting dietary fiber that are also beneficial that haven't yet been identified. You can't just borrow some *Faecalibacterium prausnitzii* from your lean vegan friend while you continue to eat cheeseburgers every day, although it's not so much the presence of cheeseburgers that's the problem—it's the absence of enough high-fiber foods.

When in Doubt, Eat More Fiber

A healthy diet that can protect you from chronic diseases and viruses is all about what you're missing, and most people in developed countries are missing fiber—not fiber from granola bars, muffins, bread, or breakfast cereal, but unprocessed fiber from vegetables, fruits, beans, whole grains, nuts, and seeds in their natural state. That type of fiber is called "indigestible" because it's not fully broken down in your intestines and creates prebiotic food for your gut bacteria to ferment and make SCFAs out of. Many studies have noted an inverse correlation between indigestible fiber intake and levels of pro-inflammatory markers, confirming that what you feed your gut bacteria matters greatly. Adding in large amounts of indigestible plant fiber is literally one of your most effective anti-viral strategies.

Fiber is the extraordinary ingredient that will strengthen your gut shield by increasing levels of bacteria like *Faecalibacterium prausnitzii*, which in turn churn out large amounts of SCFAs, which then guide and set your immune system to a Goldilocks "just right" response. This is synergy that cannot be hacked but can be reinforced every day by the food choices you make. In the Anti-Viral Gut Plan in the third part of this book I'll give you clear directions for how to simply and tastily maximize the amount of indigestible plant fiber you're consuming.

By now you're probably convinced that eating large amounts of indigestible plant fiber is a great idea. But just in case you need another nudge, let me tell you about what happens in your gut when you don't get enough fiber: your gut bacteria start to feed on the protective mucus lining of your gut, which disrupts one of your most important physical barriers that's designed to keep deadly viruses safely away from your internal organs. In a recent study from the University of Michigan Medical School, Eric Martens and colleagues fed mice three different diets: one was high in fiber, the other was fiber-free, and the third was mixed: high-fiber chow and fiber-free chow on alternating days. The high-fiber diet group had a healthy protective mucus lining, while those on the fiber-free diet had a dramatically diminished mucus layer. The alternating high-fiber diet wasn't enough to keep the gut healthy, either: these mice had a mucus layer about half the thickness of mice on the daily high-fiber diet, suggesting that eating high-fiber foods every other day is still not enough to protect you. Martens and his colleagues also found that mice on the daily high-fiber diet consumed fewer calories and were slimmer than those on the fiber-free diet—results also confirmed by multiple studies in humans that show the superiority of a plant-based diet for maintaining a healthy weight.

NURTURE IS ON YOUR SIDE

This idea that how you live (nurture), not your genes (nature), decides your fate is one that will come up again and again throughout this book. It's a remarkable message of optimism, especially now as we face current and future viral threats, to know that simple changes that are within your reach can have a profound impact on your risk of getting sick and your ability to recover fully. This protective effect isn't random. It's not just good or bad luck—it's predictable and preventable. Predictable because high levels of fiber equal high levels of protective microbes and metabolites. Preventable because those high levels mean less severe (or no) viral illness.

. . . . .

Now let's take a look at another significant digestive health variable, this time the lining of your gut, which can protect you when it's intact or render you more susceptible to viral attack when it's not.

To view the scientific references cited in this chapter, please visit
drrobynnechutkan.com/anti-viral-gut-references.

5

Breached: The Leaky Gut

All disease begins in the gut.

—Hippocrates

In the early 1990s, researchers did a series of experiments that involved taking bacteria normally found in the digestive tracts of rats and injecting those same bacteria into the wall of the rodents' colons. The results were more dramatic than anyone expected—this simple maneuver of transferring bacteria just beyond the razor-thin lining of the gut created severe inflammation not just in the bowel itself but systemically throughout the body. The experiments highlighted the importance of the gut epithelial barrier for separating the contents of the digestive tract from the rest of the body, and what could happen when it was inappropriately breached.

We've seen biopsy and autopsy evidence of infection in the liver, heart, kidneys, bladder, and brain in some people with severe viral illnesses. But why do physical barriers like your gut lining limit viral invasion in some otherwise healthy people, while allowing unfettered passage (with dire consequences) in others? What causes those barrier breaches and how can we prevent them so that if we do get infected with a virus, we're able to contain and limit the damage?

IN VERSUS OUT

When you eat, food enters your mouth and eventually the products of your streamlined digestive system come out the other end. But during that voyage, the food is never really inside your body; it's in your digestive tract—a hollow tube that runs from your mouth to your anus. In order to get inside your body, the contents of your gut have to be absorbed through your intestinal lining, a thin membrane made up of a single layer of epithelial cells that serves as a selective barrier to entry. That membrane is critically important because it's the only thing protecting you from the outside world of potentially harmful viruses, bacteria, and other toxins that you ingest every day. Like a seasoned bouncer at an exclusive club who keeps out the drunk and disorderly, your gut lining has to be very selective about what it lets in—and out. Nutrients and other essential compounds are supposed to make their way in, while waste matter from cells makes its way out.

Absorption and excretion aren't the only things going on across your gut lining—it's also a critical border zone, with your immune system on one side regulating responses, and trillions of microbes on the other guiding that immune response and helping to keep the lining healthy. The interaction between the two is one of the most complex relationships in your body. When your gut lining becomes damaged, this relationship breaks down, and the drunk and disorderly ooze through into your bloodstream, an event known as leaky gut that has serious ramifications for your immune system and your ability to defend yourself from viruses.

WHAT CAUSES LEAKS?

Five factors—diet, bacterial imbalance, medications, stress, and inflammation—play a big role in increasing your intestinal permeability and creating a leaky gut. As you'll see, there's a lot of overlap between the things that can damage your microbiome—things we learned about in the previous chapter—and those that also prove problematic for your intestinal lining. That's not surprising, since the two conditions often coexist.

Some specifics:

- Eating a diet high in refined sugar, processed foods, preservatives, and chemicals has been associated with leaky gut, and in some people, so has regular consumption of gluten, a protein found in wheat, rye, and barley. Excessive alcohol use can also damage your intestinal lining.

- An intact gut lining requires the right balance of gut bacteria, so dysbiosis, an imbalance between beneficial and harmful species that also includes overgrowth of microbes that can damage the epithelial barrier, is one of the leading causes of increased intestinal permeability.

- Medications such as aspirin and nonsteroidal anti-inflammatories (NSAIDs) are known to cause ulceration in the gastrointestinal (GI) tract, which are literally small holes in the lining. Acid blockers that change the pH of the gut, steroids that alter the intestinal milieu, and antibiotics that kill off essential good bacteria are all associated with both dysbiosis and increased intestinal permeability.

- Stress—and the heightened inflammation that follows it— triggers growth of pathogenic bacteria that can more easily bridge your gut lining. Chronic stress also weakens your immune system, affecting your ability to fight off invading pathogens and worsening the symptoms of leaky gut.

- Gastrointestinal inflammatory conditions like ulcerative colitis, Crohn's, and celiac disease are all associated with leaky gut. Radiation and chemotherapy can also cause chronic inflammation in the digestive tract, which can lead to damage to the lining and leaky gut.

WHAT DO LEAKS CAUSE?

Your immune system is a complicated network of cells and organs that protects you from germs and other harmful substances. A crucial function of this network is the ability to distinguish between what's a normal part of your body and what's a foreign invader. When substances leak through your intestinal membrane, they're identified by your immune system as foreign and a cascade of events ensues, resulting in inflammation in various parts of your body that can lead to a wide variety of nonspecific symptoms, including bloating, cramps, fatigue, food sensitivities, flushing, achy joints, headache, rashes, and more—some of the same systemic effects the researchers noted in those early gut barrier experiments in the 1990s.

In addition to stimulating an immune response, a leak can compromise your body's receipt of nutrients. With leaky gut, poor absorption of nutrients often develops as a result of damage to the villi—the fingerlike projections in your small intestine responsible for absorbing nutrients—resulting in deficiencies and malnutrition even if you're eating a relatively healthy diet. Multiple food sensitivities are another hallmark of leaky gut, as your immune system reacts to the incompletely digested particles of protein and fat that leak through your intestinal wall.

Despite all the problems it causes, leaky gut can be a challenging diagnosis to make. While colon cancer, polyps, gallstones, hepatitis, and ulcers cause changes in the GI tract you can detect with an endoscope, ultrasound, or blood test, a diagnosis like leaky gut is much more nuanced. Although there are some commercially available tests for diagnosing increased intestinal permeability, none are super specific or reliable. As a result, there's a fair amount of skepticism in the mainstream medical community about the legitimacy of leaky gut as a diagnosis, although as evidence mounts that this is indeed a real and recognizable condition, opinions are changing. The recent pandemic has contributed to that shift in thinking, since there's now clear evidence that leaky gut contributes to worse outcomes in viral infections. Let's take a closer look.

THE PROBLEMS WITH A WEAKENED CRITICAL BARRIER

People with underlying medical conditions like high blood pressure, diabetes, and obesity face a higher risk of severe viral infections, and so do older people, with the elderly most vulnerable to serious complications and a likelihood of hospitalization and death. Both of these factors—advanced age and chronic conditions—have a well-known association with altered gut barrier function, allowing pathogens easier access to critical internal organs.

Microbiologist Heenam Kim, from Korea University's Laboratory for Human-Microbial Interactions, analyzed data connecting gut health and prognosis in viral illnesses. His findings confirmed that gut dysfunction like leaky gut worsens the severity of infection by allowing the virus access to blood vessels, liver, kidney, and heart through the digestive tract. Other researchers have also found that with severe viral infections, there is a steep increase in permeability of the gut epithelial tight junctions, consistent with a loss of the intestinal barrier function. This is frequently accompanied by an increase in the protein zonulin, a known marker for increased intestinal (and brain) permeability.

And with COVID, we have specific evidence of this mechanism at work: since the early reports of a severe COVID-related condition, researchers have been trying to figure out what drives the inflammation in multisystem inflammatory syndrome (MIS), an immune response to the virus that involves multiple organs, including the gastrointestinal tract, heart, lungs, kidneys, brain, and skin and can occur in both children and adults. GI symptoms like diarrhea, vomiting, and loss of appetite are common in MIS, and that's not surprising, since viral RNA is present in the stool of people with MIS. But people with MIS also have something else going on: antigens to the virus and elevated zonulin levels in their blood. This strongly suggests that the virus is crossing from the gut to the bloodstream and causing MIS, and that the process is driven by an increase in intestinal permeability. These recent findings validate what the research from a few decades ago also demonstrated: the gut epithelial barrier plays a critical role in providing protection from pathogens, and breaching it can have serious consequences.

PATCHING THE HOLES

What can you do to prevent your gut from leaking and suffering all the potential consequences, including worse outcomes from viruses? Short-chain fatty acids (SCFAs) to the rescue. SCFAs, like butyric, propionic, and acetic acids, play a pivotal role in maintaining the integrity of your gut barrier, so it's not surprising that the depletion of *Faecalibacterium prausnitzii* and other bacteria that produce SCFAs is one of the main causes of a leaky gut. If your levels of this essential bacteria are low, your intestinal permeability is likely to be high. That makes you more vulnerable to infection by allowing viruses to seep through your leaky gut lining and gain access to your internal organs.

How many people worried about coming down with complications from a viral illness are aware that something as simple as not eating enough fiber or consuming too much sugary processed foods puts you at risk for a leaky gut and severe complications? Just eating a salad every day, as well as some of the high-inulin prebiotic foods like asparagus, leeks, and garlic, which feed your good bacteria, can help you boost your population of *Faecalibacterium prausnitzii*, increase your SCFAs, tighten up the protective junctions in your gut lining, and significantly improve your outcome from viral infection. It really is that straightforward.

ACUTE ON TOP OF CHRONIC

Unfortunately, not everyone eats this way. Lisa was a patient of mine who was an extremely picky eater in childhood. Her staple diet was McDonald's chicken nuggets and fries up until her mid-twenties. In her early thirties, she traveled to Mexico and came down with a severe case of viral gastroenteritis that led to five days in the hospital, two different potent IV antibiotics (since initially they suspected the cause was bacterial), plus round-the-clock Motrin for cramps and fever. She was discharged on an additional two weeks of broad-spectrum antibiotics, and a few weeks later started having diarrhea and bloating. Two months after her initial illness, she was prescribed two more rounds of antibiotics for a resistant urinary tract infection, and then another antibiotic for a sinus infection that wasn't getting better on its own. Her diarrhea worsened and she developed a vaginal yeast infection, and—as if that wasn't enough—she started having headaches and joint pain. That's when she came to see me, wondering whether I knew of some pill or supplement that could get her back to her previous baseline of relatively good health.

Although Lisa hadn't taken a lot of antibiotics before her trip to Mexico, she'd been on acid blockers for several years for heartburn and had a long history of daily ibuprofen use—both major risk factors for increasing intestinal permeability. An acute infection like gastroenteritis,

whether bacterial, viral, or parasitic in origin, can disrupt your microbiome, and in Lisa's case, the boatload of antibiotics that followed
were likely the triggering event that led to acute damage to her gut
lining. We know that a leaky gut is often accompanied by dysbiosis,
and there's lots of overlap between the two, which makes it difficult to
draw a straight line from clear cause to specific symptom. Lisa's diarrhea, bloating, yeast overgrowth, joint pain, headaches, and frequent
infections were likely a combination of chronic damage to both her
gut lining and her microbiome from years of acid blockers and ibuprofen, exacerbated and compounded by her acute infection and the
heavy load of antibiotics. Not only was her intestinal membrane severely compromised, but she was also missing tons of microbes!

I explained to Lisa that the most important part of getting her
better wasn't adding more medications or supplements, but actually
steering clear of all the drugs—prescription and over the counter—
that had helped to create the damage. Her symptoms eventually resolved a few months after stopping the antibiotics, acid blockers, and
NSAIDs, with the help of a major dietary overhaul that included lots
of high-fiber and fermented foods (and a startling absence of chicken
nuggets), plus a glutamine supplement that may or may not have been
helping, but wasn't harmful and that she was interested in taking.

Lisa's experience highlights how a background of seemingly benign
risk factors like acid blockers, NSAIDs, and a suboptimal diet—all of
which she wasn't even aware were a problem—can predispose you to
leaky gut after an acute event like an infection, especially if you end
up receiving additional courses of antibiotics. Fortunately, Lisa made
a complete recovery, but my gastroenterology practice is full of people
who have been diagnosed with "post-infectious irritable bowel syndrome" after an acute episode of gastroenteritis, and whose gut is
never the same because of the increase in intestinal permeability.

REMOVE, REPLACE, RESTORE

There's no miracle antidote for a leaky gut (and beware of untested supplement "cures"), but there are definitely things you can do to help heal inflammation and restore the integrity of your gut lining. These solutions focus on *removing* offending agents, *replacing* good bacteria in your gut, and *restoring* a damaged intestinal lining. I'll explain the specific steps involved in the Anti-Viral Gut Plan.

It's not just exposure to viruses that's the problem; it's when they manage to gain access to your insides and impact the function of your organs. Your gut lining is one of those critical internal barriers to viral penetration that can protect you from their widespread and potentially fatal systemic effects. In the next chapter, we're going to explore the impact of external factors like stress and lack of sleep, and the profound effect changes in body weight can have on your response to viruses. The good news is that these are all vulnerabilities within your control—and once you learn more about how dramatically they alter your risk, you'll be more motivated than ever to pull the blinds, do a little meditating, and consider whether now might be the time to get in the best shape of your life.

To view the scientific references cited in this chapter, please visit

drrobynnechutkan.com/anti-viral-gut-references.

6

Additional Vulnerabilities

A good laugh and a long sleep are the best cures in the doctor's book.

—Irish proverb

We've only recently come to accept that mental health is in fact part of overall health and that what's going on in your head is very much connected to the rest of your body, including (and especially) your gut and immune system. Our culture prides itself on high productivity, and all-nighters and minimal sleep are often regarded as badges of honor, despite the toll they can take on our well-being. While you can't always tell if someone is stressed or sleep-deprived just by looking at them, you can assess whether they're overweight or obese. But while we tend to focus on the optics of weight, it's the profound internal effects excess weight has on our bodily functions we should be concerned about. If you struggle with your weight, feel stressed out, or need to get more rest, you may worry about being perceived as weak. But the irony is that paying close attention to these factors actually makes you stronger, particularly when it comes to resisting viruses. Let's explore the role of sleep, stress, and weight on your ability to fight viruses.

LACK OF SHUT-EYE

Neuroscientist Matthew Walker describes a global real-life experiment in sleep loss that occurs every year among 1.6 billion people in seventy different countries. It's called daylight savings time (DST). When we lose an hour of sleep each spring by pushing the clocks forward, hospitals report a 24 percent spike in heart attack visits the next day. And when we turn the clocks back in the fall and gain an extra hour of sleep, heart attack visits drop by 21 percent the next day. That's how sensitive your body is to sleep. Literally no aspect of your physiology escapes the effects of sleep deprivation, and short sleep actually predicts short life. But does it also predict increased susceptibility to viruses?

What Happens When You Sleep?

When you sleep, it may seem as though you're not really doing anything, but nothing could be further from the truth. During sleep, your brain and body are busy organizing nerve cells, establishing neural pathways, regulating hormones, repairing cells, and clearing out toxins. You're actually learning new skills while you're asleep, and that's also the time when your brain processes memories, gaining insights and finding solutions to problems you weren't able to while you were awake. That's why when you're struggling to figure something out, it can be so helpful to "sleep on it" (some of the best parts of this book emerged while I was sleeping).

Elite athletes point to sleep as a vital part of their recovery that's critical to maintaining high performance levels. In Anders Ericsson's book *Peak,* where he studies the science of expertise, he reports that for world-class violinists, sleep is the second most important factor in improving, after practice itself.

And When You Don't?

Sleep helps you learn, grow, and thrive—but only when you're getting enough of it. Babies and toddlers need a lot of sleep (ideally, much more time asleep than awake) so they can process and consolidate all the new things they're learning every day. School-age kids require between nine and eleven hours, teens should aim for eight to ten hours, and adults need between seven and nine. The Centers for Disease Control and Prevention (CDC) says adults should get a minimum of seven hours of sleep every night, but only two out of three Americans actually achieve that.

In addition to cognitive and systemic effects that occur when you don't get enough sleep, your risk for contracting viral infections skyrockets, too. Just how much of a risk factor are we talking about? A study published in *The BMJ* found that people who are regularly sleep deprived have an 88 percent greater risk of contracting viral infections. The researchers noted that every one-hour increase in the amount of time spent asleep at night was associated with an additional 12 percent lower odds of becoming infected. That's because sleep deprivation triggers the release of substances that cause inflammation and leads to changes in your immune system that increase susceptibility to illness. Let's explore exactly how and why this happens.

Sleep-Deprived and Sick

You've probably noticed that when you're run down and sleep-deprived, you're more susceptible to the flu or a cold. That's no coincidence. Like an overheated computer, your immune system is malfunctioning because it's not getting the sleep it needs. Sleep literally reboots your immune system, and it's a must-have requirement for it to do its job properly. While you sleep, your immune system is busy producing infection-fighting antibodies and cytokines that help protect you from invading viruses. We have real scientific evidence of that production: a 2019 study showed that people who get eight hours of sleep a night have higher levels of T cells than those who sleep less. Thus loss of sleep translates into a decreased ability to fend off viral invaders, making it harder for you to recover from an infection.

And that risk isn't just theoretical. A study published in the journal *Sleep* found that people who got at least seven hours of sleep were four times less likely to come down with a cold than those who clocked fewer than six hours, and fewer than five hours of nightly sleep (or fragmented sleep) correlated with an increased risk of coming down with pneumonia. In clinical studies where healthy adults were inoculated with rhinovirus, those with poor sleep were much more likely to get sick, and when they did, they had more symptoms.

This dramatic state of immune deficiency associated with sleep deprivation happens quickly—after just one night of poor sleep. Fewer than four hours of night sleep is correlated with a 70 percent drop in critical immune cells the next day. There is no denying that good sleep is absolutely imperative if you're trying to stay healthy and avoid coming down with a virus.

**SIGNS AND SYMPTOMS OF
CHRONIC SLEEP DEPRIVATION**
Accidents due to daytime drowsiness
Anxiety
Decreased fertility
Depressed mood
High blood pressure
Increased risk of diabetes
Increased risk of heart disease
Increased risk of infection

Irritability

Low sex drive

Memory issues

Poor balance

Shortened life expectancy

Trouble with thinking and concentration

Weakened immunity

Weight gain

SLEEP AND VACCINES

Research shows that sleep can boost your innate and acquired immune responses, and that includes responses to vaccines, too. A study from 2020, published in the *International Journal of Behavioral Medicine,* found that the flu vaccine was more effective in people who got sufficient sleep for the two nights prior to receiving it compared to those who were sleep-deprived. The immunologic response to the vaccine can be reduced by over 50 percent in those with partial sleep loss, compared to those with a regular sleep schedule, and the same is true for the hepatitis A and B vaccine. According to the American Academy of Sleep Medicine, getting good sleep before and after receiving the COVID vaccine could be the difference between a response that actually protects you and one that doesn't.

The Gut-Sleep Connection

Sleep profoundly affects your immune system, but your microbes in turn impact your sleep in two important ways: through regulation of hormones, and via bidirectional communication with your brain known as the gut-brain axis. So good sleep, a healthy microbiome, and an effective immune response are all connected. Let's explore that connection by taking a look at your gut bacteria's intimate involvement in the production of a critical sleep hormone.

Serotonin is sometimes referred to as the feel-good hormone because of its stabilizing effect on mood, feelings of well-being, and happiness. Serotonin is also the precursor for the sleep hormone melatonin, 90 percent of which is manufactured by your gut bacteria from the amino acid tryptophan. A damaged or unhealthy microbiome can affect serotonin production, which can in turn affect melatonin production, and as you'll see, melatonin is critical for falling asleep.

How critical? Your circadian rhythm, your body's natural, internal process that regulates your sleep-wake cycle, relies on melatonin to do its job. As it gets darker, your eyes sense less light and send a message to your brain via your optic nerve that night is coming. In response, your brain increases melatonin secretion to make you sleepy. That's why darkness—and the melatonin it induces—is so essential for falling asleep. In the morning, the opposite happens: as light increases, melatonin secretion decreases, and you wake up. Gut bacteria's involvement in serotonin production ties your microbiome into the sleep equation: low microbial diversity in your gut leads to low serotonin and melatonin production, and poor sleep. That in turn leads to increased susceptibility to viral illness because of the effect of that poor sleep on your immune system. High gut diversity and richness are associated with high serotonin and melatonin production, improved sleep quality, and an intact immune response.

In addition to those important hormonal cues, there are communication pathways between your gut and your brain that involve key signals being passed back and forth. That bidirectional chatter between the two systems impacts your stress response, your mood, your appetite—and your sleep patterns. The communication between the two organs is heavily influenced by the health of your gut bacteria. An imbalanced or dysbiotic microbiome produces altered metabolites, some of which are inflammatory to the brain. These "neuroinflammatory" products can travel from your gut to your brain and disrupt the chemical signaling required to maintain a healthy sleep profile. The negative effect of those gut-derived metabolites on your sleep puts you at increased risk for viral infection. And of course the converse is true: a healthy microbiome leads to healthy gut-brain communication pathways that enhance rather than disrupt your sleep, ensuring that your immune system is rebooted and ready to do battle.

Sleep Interventions

If you've been searching for the secret sauce that will help you live, look, and feel better, as well as dramatically improve your resilience to viruses, you need only get horizontal and close your eyes to find it. Whether you're trying to optimize your immune system and prevent infection, enhance your response to anti-viral vaccines, or find relief from post-viral symptoms like brain fog and fatigue, sleep is the must-have instrument in your toolbox. And since the health of your microbiome influences your serotonin levels, which in turn affect your melatonin production and your likelihood of getting a good night's sleep, good guts predict good sleep.

Just as disordered sleep affects every aspect of your health and well-being, restoring sleep is just as impactful in making your life better, and that can happen in as few as four days of good sleep hygiene. Imagine what it would feel like to open your eyes in the morning after a solid night's rest, feeling refreshed, energized, and optimistic; to experience a brighter mood, heightened cognition, better memory, a body that moves with more ease, and improvements in every organ, from your brain to your ankle joints, and everything in between; and to know that your entire body's virus-fighting machinery is well-rested and ready to defend you. I'll take you through all the different methods of sleep restoration, including bedtime routine, sleep environment, diet, mind-body practices, supplements, and medications in the Anti-Viral Gut Plan.

Stressed About Not Sleeping?

Fewer than seven hours of sleep per night on a regular basis essentially creates a fight-or-flight state, with increased stress hormones and the release of adrenaline. The irony is that the more we stress about not sleeping or getting sick, the likelier this is to happen. Why? Because stress isn't just in your head—it's also very much in your body.

STRESS TEST

I get really stressed out by snakes. If one slithered into the room right now, a few things would happen. I'd start breathing really fast, my heart rate would increase, my blood pressure would go up, I'd become sweaty and clammy, I'd bolt out of the room, and I'd break out in goose bumps. (I can make my heart rate go up a little just by thinking about the time I was using the bathroom in a barn and looked up to see a big yellow snake in the rafters peering down at me.) All these physical manifestations can occur, just based on your emotions.

Acute versus Chronic Stress

Despite the physical, behavioral, and emotional changes it can cause, not all stress is bad. Short bursts of acute stress can actually produce adaptive advantages in your body that many times can save you from danger (think: avoiding snakes!). That's very different from the effects of chronic stress, which ironically puts you in danger by weakening your immune system. With acute stress, your adrenal glands churn out cortisol, the stress hormone, as well as the fight-or-flight hormones epinephrine and norepinephrine, to keep you alert and ready to spring into action. These hormones help you access quick sources of energy so you can deal with the stressor at hand. During periods of acute stress, cells in your innate immune system are activated and increase their patrol for infectious pathogens, so that alive-awake-alert-enthusiastic feeling that acute stress elicits can actually help you evade viruses and give you a survival advantage.

But once the threat or danger passes, your relaxation response is supposed to kick in to get you back to a normal, mellow state. Unfortunately, dealing with modern life (not to mention a pandemic) keeps many of us constantly revved up, in a chronic fight-or-flight state that works against us and actually makes us more vulnerable. With chronic stress, your body produces a continuous acute stress response, which leads to changes that can drive up your blood pressure, damage your arteries and heart, interfere with your ability to think clearly, decrease your thyroid function and bone density, increase your blood sugar, cause inflammation in multiple organs, and lead to belly fat associated with metabolic syndrome (a cluster of conditions that increase the risk of heart disease, stroke, and diabetes) and a higher chance of dying. Think running at high speeds for long periods of time, versus cruising along at a moderate pace, and what that can do your body over time.

It's important to be familiar with the multiple ways chronic stress can manifest itself, so you can recognize when it's occurring and take steps to try to ameliorate it. It's especially important now, given the threat of viral pandemics that will likely become part of our daily existence (which is itself stress-inducing), plus the fact that being stressed out puts you at a much higher risk for becoming infected.

SIGNS AND SYMPTOMS OF CHRONIC STRESS

PHYSICAL

- Stiff or tense muscles, especially in the neck or shoulders
- Headaches
- Shakiness or tremors
- Loss of interest in sex

- Weight gain or loss
- Restlessness
- Physical discomfort
- Altered breathing pattern

BEHAVIORAL
- Procrastination
- Grinding teeth
- Difficulty completing work assignments
- Changes in the amount of alcohol or food you consume
- Sleeping too much or too little

EMOTIONAL
- Crying
- Overwhelming sense of tension or pressure
- Trouble relaxing
- Nervousness
- Quick temper
- Depression
- Poor concentration
- Trouble remembering things
- Loss of sense of humor

Stressed Out and Sick

Long before the pandemic there was already lots of evidence linking stress to increased susceptibility to viral infections. A classic study at Carnegie Mellon University showed that the risk for the common cold was proportional to the degree of stress in a person's life, and a subsequent study showed that people who had chronic stress due to life events like unemployment or interpersonal problems for at least one month were much more likely to get the common cold than those who had shorter durations of stress. In research published in *Proceedings of the National Academy of Sciences,* 276 healthy adults were exposed to a virus that causes colds and then monitored in quarantine for five days. Those who indicated they were under chronic stress were twice as likely to get sick, and more likely to produce cytokines that trigger inflammation. A study published in *Annals of Internal Medicine* looked at adults fifty and older and found that those with a daily stress-reducing routine like exercise or mindfulness meditation were less likely to get sick with a respiratory infection than subjects in a control group, and if they did get sick, they missed fewer days of work.

Chronic stress doesn't just increase your susceptibility to new viral infections, it also makes you more vulnerable to reactivation or progression of ones you already have. Some viruses are never fully cleared from your body; instead, they go into a latent inactive state. Common examples in humans include herpes simplex, which causes oral and genital herpes; varicella zoster, which is responsible for chickenpox and shingles; and Epstein-Barr virus, which is associated with mono. The problem if you have one of these viruses is that in times of stress, when your immune system is suppressed and not able to protect you as well, the virus can reactivate and start reproducing, taking over, killing cells, and causing a flare-up of symptoms like cold sores and genital ulcers, painful shingles lesions, or knocking you off your feet with a relapse of mono. Stress can even cause people infected with HIV to experience a quicker progression to AIDS. A University of North Carolina–Chapel Hill study found that men with HIV progressed to AIDS faster if they had chronic stress in their lives, and for each increased stressful event, the risk for AIDS progression doubled.

These links between stress and your risk for viral infection aren't just theoretical concerns. They're real, legitimate, and compelling explanations for why when you're stressed you're more likely to get sick and have a more difficult time recovering. I see examples of this playing out every day in my medical practice. People come in tense and worried about getting sick, looking for advice on the ideal probiotic or what supplement to take. They're surprised when I tell them that their stressed-out state is the main thing that's putting them at risk, and what they really need isn't a probiotic or supplement, but to learn how to relax and stress less. Take a patient of mine, Joe, who's a lawyer. Every time he had a big case, Joe would get a severe herpes outbreak. He would take the anti-viral medication acyclovir for the flare-ups, and while it helped shorten the length of outbreaks, it gave him nausea and stomach pain and didn't prevent future episodes. A regular meditation practice finally helped him break the cycle and he hasn't needed an anti-viral prescription in years. (We'll talk more about stress-relieving strategies in Chapter 10.)

In almost every study looking at viral-related health outcomes, including COVID prognosis, chronic stress is considered a significant risk factor for poor outcomes. And it's an important one to pay attention to, because unlike some other risk factors like age or cardiovascular status, chronic stress is inherently modifiable. But how exactly does chronic stress make you more vulnerable to getting sick? Sustained secretion of stress hormones weakens your adaptive immune system, suppressing white blood cells and leaving you less able to produce antibodies and more susceptible to infections. Chronic stress also causes release of pro-inflammatory cytokines, which may contribute to a potentially fatal cytokine storm if you have a viral infection.

What's Your Gut Got to Do with It?

As described in Chapter 1, most of your immune system is located in your gastrointestinal (GI) tract, and as we just learned, stress can have devastating effects on your immune response. But there's an even more direct connection between stress and your gut. Chances are you've had the sensation of butterflies in your stomach right before a big event or before you followed your "gut instinct" when making a tough decision. Those "nerves" in your gut are real—you actually have a second nervous system in your gut called the enteric nervous system, and it has about seven times as many nerve cells as your spinal cord. It's not surprising, then, that your gut plays a big role in your stress response. At the same time, stress can substantially and rapidly influence what's going on in your gut, including which of your gut microbes thrive and which ones perish.

Stress isn't just bad for you; it's bad for your gut bacteria, too. High levels of stress can affect the amount of mucus production in your digestive tract, which changes the composition, diversity, and amount of bacteria growing in your gut. Not only is there less species variation with stress, but the numbers of potentially harmful bacteria rise, too, which makes you more susceptible to infection.

Catecholamines are neurotransmitter hormones that help your body respond to stress and prepare for fight-or-flight reactions. Your adrenal glands churn out large amounts of catecholamines like epinephrine (adrenaline), norepinephrine (noradrenaline), and dopamine as a reaction to stress, and those catecholamines can increase levels of harmful gut bacteria ten-thousand-fold and intensify their infectiousness in fewer than twenty-four hours. These more pathogenic bacteria can crowd out beneficial species and lead to dysbiosis, increasing your risk for viral infection. In a well-known experiment looking at the impact of academic stress on college students, beneficial lactic acid bacterial levels were measured and found to be much lower during high stress periods like exams, and higher when the students were under less stress, validating the link between stress and gut flora activity.

Another way that stress impacts your digestive tract and increases your susceptibility to viruses is through its effects on your gut lining. As we have discussed, that lining is one of the most important physical barriers to viral entry, and stress can compromise its barrier function by increasing the permeability of the lining, making it easier for viruses to penetrate and infect your other organs.

A Learned Response

You may not be able to change a stressful living or work situation, but you can learn to change your response to it, and altering that stress response can significantly improve your resiliency to viruses. Given the impact of stress on the immune system, it's no wonder that people who worry and stress a lot about getting sick often do get sick more frequently.

Gloria is another patient who I first met when she was in high school. She graduated summa cum laude from college with a degree in biochemistry and was doing basic science research over the summer, plus working full-time in a doctor's office and finishing her medical school applications. The last year was challenging for Gloria. In addition to getting COVID, she ended up with two episodes of viral gastroenteritis and the flu. Everything started while she was studying for her MCATs, and as she got closer to the medical school application deadlines and interview season, her health really declined. Granted, her job in a doctor's office meant there were plenty of germs floating around, but exposure was only part of the story.

Gloria is an obsessive perfectionist who tackles every task like her life depends on it. It's gotten her far academically, and she's the kind of team member employers dream about, but it's come at a price. Gloria suffers from GI distress that was diagnosed as irritable bowel syndrome when she was a young teen.

After her second bout of gastroenteritis, I finally convinced Gloria that something had to give, and she agreed to wrap up her research project and cut down her hours at the doctor's office. Not surprisingly, her immunity improved, too, and so did her cycle of frequent viral infections. Despite feeling better, Gloria wanted to know if there was something she could take to safeguard against the future stress she anticipated in medical school. But Dr. Ashwin Mehta, medical director of integrative medicine at Memorial Healthcare System, says it best: "Stress exists in the realm of the mind. Therefore, the tools that we must use in order to confront excessive stress need to also be mindfulness-based modalities."

Interventions to De-stress

Not enough sleep and too much stress seem to go hand in hand, but the good news is the solutions for one often improve the other. A 2021 publication on the neurobiology of stress confirmed that stress-reducing psychosocial interventions (that also help you sleep better), including relaxation techniques and behavioral therapy, can optimize neuroendocrine-immune responses against viral infections both during and beyond the COVID pandemic. In the Anti-Viral Gut Plan, I'll take you through some important principles of de-stressing, as well as provide you with clear direction for how to harness and utilize your virus-fighting relaxation response.

WEIGHING IN ON WEIGHT

I want to dive into a topic that can be uncomfortable for some people, and that's the subject of weight. At this moment in time, thinking deeply about what it means to be overweight or obese doesn't have anything to do with aesthetics or body shaming. It has to do with surviving viral threats that are likely going to be with us for a long time and for which excess weight can be deadly.

At Risk

We've known for over a century, since the influenza pandemic of 1918, that obesity is linked to a worse prognosis for viral infections.

The 1957–60 "Asian" and the 1968 "Hong Kong" influenza epidemics confirmed that excess weight leads to a higher mortality as well as a more prolonged duration of illness, even in the absence of other chronic conditions. With the 2009 H1N1 outbreak, people who were obese had more severe disease and a higher likelihood of hospitalization and death.

Since the SARS-CoV-2 pandemic began, several studies have reported that many of the sickest COVID patients have been people with obesity, and the vast majority—78 percent—of U.S. patients hospitalized with COVID have been overweight or obese. (The Centers for Disease Control and Prevention defines overweight as having a BMI of 25 to 29.9, and obesity as a BMI of 30 or greater.) In a large analysis of almost half a million patients published in *Obesity Reviews,* obese people infected with viruses were 113 percent more likely than people of healthy weight to land in the hospital, 74 percent more likely to be admitted to an ICU, and 48 percent more likely to die. Other studies have shown that having obesity triples your likelihood of being hospitalized for COVID and is the number one risk factor for dying from it in people under sixty-five.

Why does having excess weight put you at such high risk for complications of viral illness? The answer is a combination of anatomical, physiological, immunological, and social factors. The mechanics of obesity lead to reduced lung volume and restricted air flow, as well as blood that's "stickier" and more prone to clot, which both contribute to complications from viral illnesses. Large numbers of viral receptors in adipose (fatty) tissue, combined with fewer immune cells because of fatty infiltration of immune organs, mean more deadly disease when overweight or obese people are infected with a virus. And there's additional impaired immunity with excess weight as a result of chronic low-grade inflammation and poorer functioning of immune cells. But perhaps the most tragic association with weight and complications from viruses is avoidance or delay in seeking medical care because obesity is so stigmatized.

A Shared Problem

Two out of three adults in the United States are overweight or obese, and at the same time, the threat from viral infections is increasing. Infectious diseases are a leading cause of death, accounting for a quarter to a third of the millions of deaths that occur worldwide every year. At least thirty previously unknown viruses have been identified since 1973, including HIV, Ebola, hepatitis C, Nipah virus, and SARS-CoV-2, for which no cures are available.

This is a problem for the individual, since excess weight increases the risk of viral infections and complications for that person. But it's also a problem for our entire society, because having a large number of obese people in the population may contribute to an increase in the overall mortality rate of a viral pandemic through two main mechanisms: (1) prolonging viral shedding and (2) increasing the chances of more virulent strains appearing.

Influenza virus shedding is 42 percent longer in obese compared to lean individuals, and similar numbers have been confirmed for other viruses, including SARS-CoV-2. The obese microenvironment has a reduced and delayed capacity to produce anti-viral interferons. That delay allows more viral RNA replication to occur, which increases the chances of novel, more virulent viral strains developing. Obesity is a public health crisis for all of us, and we all, regardless of our weight, should be thinking about how we can help those who struggle with theirs. Viral pandemics emphasize the importance of collective health and immunity. When we help our neighbors improve their viral resistance, it makes us safer, too.

In order to further understand why being obese puts you at such high risk from viruses, we need to explore the connection between obesity and the microbiome, and how that relationship impacts your immune system's ability to protect you from viruses.

Disrupted

Most healthy people have a predictable ratio of the different families of gut bacteria, but in obese people, the ratios are strikingly different, and we see lower overall species diversity and richness. We can determine whether someone is lean or obese with 90 percent accuracy just from looking at that person's gut bacteria, and we can detect species in the guts of infants as young as six months old that accurately predict the development of obesity.

Microbes from obese mice—and people—are better at extracting more calories from the same food. There are a number of ways they can do this: they can slow down the transit time of food through the digestive tract, which allows for greater absorption of calories; they can influence hormones like insulin to favor more calories being deposited as fat versus used as energy; and they can ramp up or down how many extra calories they themselves consume for tissue repair or other tasks. People colonized with gut bacteria that are more efficient at breaking down food are able to absorb more calories and end up gaining more weight, while bacteria that are not as good at extracting calories are associated with leanness.

When we transplant microbes from obese mice into germ-free lean mice, they gain weight, and their fat deposition increases without any change in their diet or exercise regimen. The same experiment can be done with humans, too: researchers at Washington University in St. Louis took gut bacteria from identical twins, where one was lean and one was obese, and transplanted them into germ-free mice. Within weeks, the mice that received microbes from the obese twin became obese, and the ones who received microbes from the lean twin stayed lean, validating the concept that our microbes, not our genes, may be primarily responsible for changes in our weight.

Researchers have identified a family of bacteria called *Christensenellaceae* that are associated with being lean, and although less than 10 percent of your microbiome is genetically determined, distribution of *Christensenellaceae* seems to be inherited. Chances are you know someone from a "skinny" family where all the members are like beanpoles, regardless of their diet. Genetic leanness is a rare exception, though. The norm for the overwhelming majority of us is that what we eat and the bacteria we cultivate as a result of our diet determine our weight.

As we saw with Dr. Lionetti's study with the children from Italy and Burkina Faso, high-fat, low-fiber diets increase the abundance of microbes associated with obesity and inflammation, while high dietary fiber intake increases microbes associated with leanness and creates a richer and more diverse microbiome. What all these observations point to is that obesity is in large part a dysbiotic state, with changes in the microbiome associated with chronic inflammation. Viral infection in someone who's significantly overweight or obese represents acute on top of chronic inflammation, and as we've seen, that can be a deadly combination. But how exactly do these obesity-associated changes in the microbiome lead to worse outcomes when infected with a virus? The link is your immune system.

Impaired

Obesity increases morbidity (getting sick) and mortality (dying) from viral infections by disrupting your immune responses, and that's true even in healthy obese subjects without comorbidities, where we still see more severe disease and complications like secondary bacterial infections and blood clots. Obese people have a higher concentration of several pro-inflammatory cytokines, which are mainly produced in their adipose tissue and lead to dysregulation of the immune response, plus more cases of cytokine storm and other forms of severe inflammation and organ damage. Unfortunately, impaired immune responses also means reduced vaccine efficacy in the obese population, which, in addition to increasing the risk of infection, can also encourage the emergence of vaccine-resistant variants.

COMPLICATIONS ASSOCIATED WITH EXCESS WEIGHT

Arthritis

Back and/or joint pain

Depression

Diabetes

Difficulty sleeping

Excessive sweating

Fatigue

Gastroesophageal reflux disease (GERD)

Heart disease

Heat intolerance

High blood pressure

Infections

Shortness of breath (dyspnea)

Sleep apnea

Obesity is a complex disease with many contributing factors. Neighborhood design, availability of healthy, affordable foods and beverages, the economics of leisure, and access to safe and convenient places for physical activity can all have a profound impact on weight. Racial and ethnic disparities in obesity highlight the need to address social determinants of health such as poverty, education, and housing. This requires action at the policy and systems level to ensure that obesity prevention and management starts early, and that everyone has access to good nutrition and safe places to be physically active. As we face more viral threats, these policy changes become imperative for both individual and collective health.

Weight Interventions

If you struggle with your weight and are concerned about susceptibility to viruses, it's not all bad news. The risk of complications and death from viral infections in people with obesity may be reduced with regular exercise, even without substantial weight loss. Several studies suggest that regular physical exercise helps to balance cytokine production during a viral infection and improves your resistance to invasion. In fact, the strongest non-pharmacological intervention to improve your immune system is physical exercise. You don't have to sign up for any marathons to get its full effect: moderate aerobic exercise (brisk walking, biking, swimming, jogging) for thirty to sixty minutes most days of the week has a profound anti-inflammatory effect, improves the hormonal milieu of people with obesity, and enhances their immune response.

Small Changes That Pack a Big Punch

It's long been established that just a 10 percent reduction in body weight in people who are overweight or obese leads to improved heart health and a lower risk of diabetes and cancer, but Australian researchers showed over a decade ago that it can also bring pro-inflammatory circulating immune cells back to the levels found in lean people. What great news! A comprehensive plan and detailed instructions for how to accomplish all of this can be found in the third part of the book.

Cultivating good sleep hygiene, managing stress, and maintaining a healthy weight are all strategies that directly impact your gut's ability to keep you safe from viruses, and even small incremental improvements in them can make a big difference in your virus-fighting capabilities.

In the next chapter, we'll move past the acute phase of viral illnesses into the realm of post-viral syndromes—what many in the age of COVID have come to know as long-haul syndrome. But post-viral symptoms aren't just a problem for people infected with SARS-CoV-2. Plenty of other viruses, including hepatitis, herpes, varicella (chicken pox), Epstein-Barr virus (mono), and others, can induce chronic symptoms long after the acute illness is gone. Understanding what puts you at risk for post-viral syndromes and the mechanisms involved in why they develop is critical for making sure that if you do get infected, your symptoms are as short-lived as possible, and your recovery is swift and complete. Spoiler alert: having a healthy gut helps!

To view the scientific references cited in this chapter, please visit
drrobynnechutkan.com/anti-viral-gut-references.

7

The Long Haul

Most patients who have had an acute infection expect to pass through a variable period of convalescence before they regain their usual health. An unlucky minority recover from the symptoms of acute disease only to be assailed by a new illness; a post-infectious syndrome.

—Dr. Barbara A. Bannister, Professor of
Infectious Diseases, Royal Free Hospital UK

Liza, a longtime friend, called me a year into the pandemic to tell me she had COVID. She had some cold symptoms, a mild cough, loss of her sense of smell, no appetite, and was really tired. When I checked back in with her a few weeks later, she was still under the weather but not as congested. Smell was coming back, and while she'd initially lost about eight pounds, her weight had started to stabilize. However, she was losing something else—her hair was falling out. Every time she washed or brushed it she'd notice clumps of hair in the shower drain or in her brush bristles. By the time I saw her a couple of months after her initial infection, there was noticeable thinning and I estimated she'd lost about 25 percent of her hair.

Beyond her hair loss, Liza just looked different. She was a little bit thinner, but that wasn't it. She just didn't look well; she had an ashen color to her skin and was moving much more slowly than normal. She resembled some of my patients with chronic autoimmune diseases like

Crohn's and ulcerative colitis when they're having a flare-up. She was also experiencing a dramatic decrease in exercise tolerance. Some of her need to take it easy was from being out of shape from months of not getting much exercise, but her shortness of breath was more than just deconditioning. She was an avid and regular runner; we had run a marathon together a few years earlier—but now when she went out for a walk she couldn't manage even short sentences without stopping to catch her breath.

The other thing that Liza was experiencing was a strange rash all over her body. She'd been advised by her doctor to take an antihistamine for the rash, but the medication made her tired and drowsy, so she took it only at night. While the rash was bothersome, some of her other symptoms had finally started to improve: her hair had stopped shedding, and she was definitely looking better physically; her color was better, her weight was back to normal, and she didn't look as weak and debilitated. She was able to walk comfortably at a vigorous pace, and had started running again, but after half a mile at a reduced pace, she had to stop and rest. She was frustrated with the slow progress of getting back into shape: it had been half a year since her COVID infection and she still couldn't run more than a mile, which was now taking her twelve minutes to complete (including a short rest stop at the half-mile mark), instead of her usual nine.

She'd had a full cardiac and pulmonary evaluation, including a stress test and ultrasound of her heart, a CAT scan of her chest, and pulmonary function tests, and had passed everything with flying colors. Rather than reassure her, the normal test results actually added to Liza's frustration. If all the tests were normal, why didn't she *feel* normal?

What ultimately helped with Liza's exercise tolerance was resuming use of the incentive spirometer (a simple handheld device that helps you breathe more deeply and fully) I'd recommended to her for the acute infection. Back then, she was doing ten deep breaths with it a couple of times a day to keep her lungs expanded and prevent bacterial pneumonia on top of COVID, which can develop when you're spending a lot of time lying on your back and not taking deep breaths. I asked Liza to increase her frequency with the spirometer to twenty deep breaths four times a day—before each meal and at bedtime to make it easy for her to remember. Liza slowly started to increase her mileage, and although at the time I wrote this book she still wasn't back up to her normal pre-COVID runs, both her mileage and her speed were continuing to improve.

Six months after her initial infection, Liza was still plagued by the rash. She noticed that high temperatures or humid conditions seemed to cause it to flare up, and so did stress. Liza has a pretty high-powered job and sits on a lot of boards, so she has plenty of time-sensitive meetings, calls, and deadlines. I recommended that she do a few minutes of focused breath work (see Chapter 10 in the Anti-Viral Gut Plan for more details) before starting any important calls or meetings to make sure she was nice and relaxed, and this got things under enough control that she was able to decrease the antihistamine use to just a couple of times a month instead of nightly.

Her doctor checked lab work on Liza and found that she had a positive antinuclear antibody test (ANA)—a blood test that can indicate the presence of autoimmune disease and suggests that your body may be attacking its own tissues. Liza didn't know what her ANA status was before she had COVID, since nobody had previously checked it, and although her test was positive, it was at a low level consistent with what we see in about one-quarter of the general healthy population. The doctor recommended that she do a follow-up test in a year to see if the level was rising or changing in any way. We're seeing more and more evidence of COVID-induced autoimmunity based on positive blood tests like the ANA and others, and while some long-haul sufferers have a history of prior autoimmune disease, most don't. An intense area of scientific investigation right now is whether long COVID patients with blood work suggestive of autoimmunity may respond to medications used to treat autoimmune diseases like lupus. Hopefully those efforts will also include complementary therapies like changes in diet and stress reduction that we've seen can be incredibly effective for treating some of those conditions.

The truth is, we really don't know what these markers of autoimmunity mean. While we do see high levels with certain diseases, we also see people with those same diseases with perfectly normal levels, and others who are healthy with elevated levels with no explanation for why. There's no clear evidence that genetic factors predispose to long COVID, but worsening of underlying conditions, including certain autoimmune diseases for which there may be a genetic influence, is a recurring theme in many long-haulers. That's why such a big part of staying well during this and future pandemics is making sure that your baseline health is as good as possible, and that includes addressing any chronic diseases with nutrition and lifestyle tactics, in addition to (or instead of, when possible) any medication you may be prescribed. Much of what goes wrong with your body is based on what's going on in your gut, so having a healthy and balanced microbiome is a winning strategy for protecting you from both acute viral infections and their chronic sequelae.

A year after her initial infection, Liza was much closer to her pre-COVID baseline but still not completely back to normal. She'd regained her full head of hair and her sense of smell had returned. A mild version of the rash flared up every few months but lasted only a day or two. She was running faster but still slower than her previous pace and doing a little less mileage than before. Multitasking and staying focused for long periods of time still felt like a challenge, but she wasn't sure how much of that was keeping up with the changing environment at home, work, and in the world versus long COVID.

She estimated that overall she was functioning at about 80 to 90 percent of her previous level, and while she was still grieving that missing 10 to 20 percent, she was also grateful for the progress she'd made.

Liza is not alone. There have been countless cases of prolonged symptoms since the pandemic first began, and long before COVID made an appearance, many people suffered from hard-to-diagnose, vague, and seemingly unrelated symptoms after viral infections. When they were seeking medical attention, it wasn't uncommon for them to hear: "Your tests are all normal," "Your symptoms are probably due to anxiety or stress," "This will likely get better on its own, but we don't know how long it will take," or a variation on this theme. If you're dealing with chronic problems after a viral illness, this may all sound painfully familiar. Post-viral symptoms can be really puzzling, even to more holistic practitioners, and because there's not always a common thread between different symptoms, an easily identifiable cause, or reliable diagnostic tests, many end up being put into the category of "medically unexplained symptoms" or MUS, and don't get the treatment they deserve.

MEDICALLY UNEXPLAINED SYMPTOMS

MUS is a medical term used to describe people who have symptoms but no clear diagnosis. The official, more unwieldy (and just as unhelpful) term is: "persistent bodily complaints for which adequate examination does not reveal sufficiently explanatory structural or other specified pathology." Translation: we have no idea what's wrong with you. A couple of examples: someone with tingling in the hands or feet, or migraines that seem like they would be caused by problems in the nervous system, but the evaluation doesn't turn up any neurological condition, or severe fatigue without any associated conditions to explain it, like anemia, an underactive thyroid, or sleep apnea.

Doctors sometimes refer to these symptoms as "functional disorders," as in a "functional neurological disorder" or a "functional bowel disorder," to imply that no clear anatomical or physiological cause has been found. I'd be lying if I didn't admit that there's a tremendous amount of bias in the medical community about whether some of these symptoms are "real," and that's unfortunate. Just because something is currently unknown doesn't mean there's not a perfectly logical and plausible future explanation. Several twentieth-century post-viral syndromes like mono and chronic hepatitis that are now well characterized and understood started out as unexplained, and the symptoms that accompany them, such as pervasive fatigue, loss of appetite, and cognitive problems, were also initially poorly understood and often ignored.

Infectious mononucleosis was recognized in the 1880s by a Russian pediatrician, who called it idiopathic adenitis in recognition of the fact that no one knew the cause ("idiopathic") and that it involved inflammation of the lymph nodes ("adenitis"). But it wasn't until forty years later, in 1920, that physicians at Johns Hopkins described the clinical characteristics of infectious mononucleosis, including the fact that it was primarily caused by the Epstein-Barr virus (EBV), and that it involved a chronic state that could develop into a type of cancer called T cell lymphoma. And the science is still evolving: as recently as 2022, research led by the Harvard T. H. Chan School of Public Health found that prior infection with EBV dramatically increases the odds of developing multiple sclerosis, a chronic and poorly understood autoimmune disease that can cause dozens of symptoms, including vision loss, pain, fatigue, and impaired coordination. Not surprisingly, as our understanding of the microbiome—the newest and perhaps broadest-reaching frontier in medicine—grows, it turns out that many of these previously "unexplained" syndromes can be attributed to disturbances in this invisible but essential ecosystem in our gut.

Before we get into the connection between the microbiome and post-viral symptoms, let's go over what's known—and what's still a mystery—about one of the most famous post-viral syndromes of this century.

LONG COVID

Early reports from Europe at the beginning of the pandemic reported persistent symptoms in a high percentage of COVID patients discharged from the hospital—as many as 80 percent in some studies. It's now clear that persistent symptoms after COVID don't occur only in hospitalized or critically ill patients but also in people who had mild disease and were never hospitalized, and even in those who had no symptoms at all. The Centers for Disease Control and Prevention (CDC) uses the umbrella term "post-COVID conditions" to refer to all new, recurrent, or ongoing symptoms four or more weeks after initial coronavirus infection. Other commonly used terms for post-COVID symptoms include "post-acute sequelae of COVID-19 (PASC)," "long COVID," "long-haul COVID," "long-haul syndrome," "chronic COVID," and "post-acute COVID-19 syndrome (PACS)."

Long COVID can affect anyone, including children and the elderly, but most studies have found women and those who had six or more symptoms during the initial infection to be the most commonly affected. Exactly how commonly long COVID occurs varies dramatically, from one in twenty patients in some studies, to around 60 percent in the over sixty-five age group and those who were hospitalized, to as high as 70 percent in those admitted to the ICU. Part of the challenge with nailing down the prevalence is that the diagnostic criteria also vary dramatically. If you look at studies that count "any symptom," the numbers are much higher than those that rely on a constellation of characteristic features, and while some people experience only one symptom, others may have several. Symptoms can range from mild to debilitating, and can interfere with school, work, or even doing simple household chores.

Because COVID can affect the function of multiple organs, long COVID is associated with a wide range of symptoms, too, including respiratory, neurological, cardiac, gastrointestinal, musculoskeletal, and psychological problems, among others. Some of the most commonly reported symptoms include fatigue, shortness of breath, chest pain, loss of smell, and "brain fog"—a mental state characterized by memory problems, confusion, and difficulty concentrating. Although there are now over two hundred different symptoms associated with long COVID, here are some of the most common:

- Abdominal pain
- Anxiety
- Brain fog (difficulty concentrating, sense of confusion or disorientation)
- Chest pain or discomfort
- Cough
- Depression
- Diarrhea
- Diminished appetite
- Dizziness
- Earache, hearing loss, and/or ringing in ears (tinnitus)
- Fatigue
- Hair loss
- Headache

- Insomnia
- Joint pain
- Low-grade intermittent fever
- Memory loss
- Muscle aches and pain/weakness
- Nausea
- Persistent loss of smell and/or taste
- Post-traumatic stress disorder (PTSD)
- Rapid or irregular heartbeat (palpitations)
- Rashes
- Shortness of breath
- Sore throat

As you can see from the list, most of these symptoms can't be confirmed with a simple test, and a diagnosis of long COVID is typically made based on a patient's history of infection and by ruling out other possible causes. The fact that we aren't entirely sure about all the mechanisms that lead to long COVID adds to the diagnostic uncertainty and makes it more challenging to come up with effective treatments. That being said, there's a lot we do know and are continuing to find out, and many of these contributing factors are also behind other post-viral syndromes. Let's review what some of the recent groundbreaking science tells us about the origins of long COVID.

What the Research Shows

With such a long list of symptoms, it can be challenging to pin down precisely what the risk factors are for long COVID, but scientists from Seattle did just that. In a study published in the journal *Cell* in 2022, they identified the most significant risk factors for developing long COVID. The top three contenders included the presence of autoantibodies in about 60 percent (like my friend Liza had), but with no evidence of autoimmune disease in the majority. Reactivation of Epstein-Barr virus, which initially affects about 90 percent of the population but normally remains dormant after initial infection, was also a risk factor, suggesting some sort of immune dysregulation that results in failure to keep EBV in check. The presence of genetic material from SARS-CoV-2 in the bloodstream was a third risk factor, confirming what we already know about the importance of epithelial barriers for controlling the spread of the virus to other parts of the body.

Another landmark study that has contributed greatly to our understanding of the mechanisms behind long COVID was also published in 2022 in the journal *Gut*. Researchers prospectively followed 106 patients with COVID from the time of their initial illness until six months after. They found a whopping 76 percent of the patients had post-COVID symptoms, most commonly fatigue, poor memory, and hair loss. What's fascinating about this study is that it showed clear (and predictable) abnormalities in the microbiome of the long COVID patients: higher levels of undesirable pathogenic species and lower levels of our old friend *Faecalibacterium prausnitzii*, the latter of which are associated with high-fiber intake, a healthy microbiome, and a balanced immune response. The study found specific microbiome abnormalities that correlated with specific symptoms in the patients with long COVID: ongoing respiratory symptoms correlated with an increase in opportunistic gut bacteria, while neuropsychiatric symptoms and fatigue were correlated with an increase in hospital-acquired gut pathogens. Overall, bacteria like *F. prausnitzii* and *Bifidobacterium*, which produce short-chain fatty acids (SCFAs), were inversely correlated with the likelihood of having long COVID, providing us with a clear path forward for addressing post-viral symptoms through paying attention to what's going on in the gut.

THE CENTRAL ROLE OF THE GUT

As a gastroenterologist, I don't find it surprising that the gut plays such a central role in both acute and chronic viral infections. Just think about where your digestive tract is located—it's in the center of your body. Your gut is the engine whose critical supply of nutrients and trillions of worker-bee microbes interact with your other bodily systems, and your gut health can greatly influence their function—or malfunction. Just imagine if your car engine stopped working. Would you still be able to drive it without serious limitations and consequences? Even if the headlights, brakes, and steering still worked, how far down the road would you get with a broken-down engine? That's why the gut is such an important connector of a lot of these symptoms, and as you'll see, it also plays a role in many post-viral causation theories.

There's a lot we're still learning about how viruses like SARS-CoV-2 and EBV cause chronic symptoms after the acute illness is over, but one of the things that's clear is that dysbiosis can be a major contributor. Let's dive a little deeper into the link between a messed-up microbiome and post-viral symptoms.

Immune-Mediated Inflammation

SARS and MERS left some people debilitated for months or even years after their acute infection, with symptoms similar to what we're seeing with long COVID. The virus was no longer active, but it triggered an inflammatory response in the body that caused persistent symptoms. We've seen similarly high levels of inflammation with long COVID. Researchers in Europe did MRI imaging of the hearts of one hundred recently recovered COVID patients and found 60 percent had ongoing heart inflammation, as well as symptoms like shortness of breath and chest pain that weren't related to preexisting conditions or the initial severity of their infection. There is mounting evidence that the culprit for these and other symptoms isn't the virus itself but rather the immune system's overzealous response to it.

To refresh your memory on immune equilibrium, let's revisit how and why things go awry. Gut bacteria normally regulate your immune response, making sure your reaction to viral infection is robust enough to clear the virus, but not so aggressive that you end up damaging your own organs. With dysbiosis, that regulation is lost, paving the way for an overblown response that can persist long after the acute infection is over and can affect many different parts of your body. Immune-mediated inflammation can wreak havoc on multiple different organs, including your brain, heart, kidneys, liver, skin, digestive tract, and more. SARS-CoV-2 is a very small virus, but it packs a big punch as far as the immune response to it goes, and that's especially true when your microbiome isn't in good enough health to keep that response in check.

Role of Dysbiosis

Dysbiosis can be both a risk factor for infection with COVID and a result of the infection. Here's how that works: ACE-2 receptors that bind SARS-CoV-2 can also disrupt the composition of your microbiome by decreasing bacterial diversity in your gut. That disruption reduces levels of healthy bacteria and their important SCFA by-products, and that can lead to dysregulation of your immune system and an exaggerated response that drives long COVID symptoms.

When you take into account the essential role gut bacteria play, not just in your immune response but in multiple aspects of your physiology, such as synthesis of hormones and vitamins, detoxification of compounds, and digestion and absorption of nutrients, plus the well-established role of the gut-brain axis in cognition, mood, memory, and neurological function, you can start to see how these shifts in the health and balance of your microbiome induced by viral infection can translate into more systemic symptoms that can be felt throughout your body. That's why optimizing your gut health plays such an important role in limiting both the acute and the chronic impact of the virus.

To understand the role of the gut in both causation and possible treatment options for post-viral syndromes like long COVID, it's helpful to take a look at some other well-known conditions that are linked to viral infection and dysbiosis.

CHRONIC FATIGUE

Lots of comparisons have been made between long COVID and chronic fatigue syndrome, also known as myalgic encephalomyelitis/chronic fatigue syndrome (ME/CFS). One of the most important recent breakthroughs in ME/CFS research is the awareness that this is a syndrome that generally arises in the gut, not in the brain. ME/CFS has been linked to viral infections like Epstein-Barr virus and human herpesvirus 6 (HHV-6), which, like COVID, can also induce disruptions in the microbiome. Additional evidence that ME/CFS is primarily a gut-based disorder comes from researchers at Cornell, who in a study published in the journal *Microbiome* describe how they were able to correctly diagnose ME/CFS in 83 percent of patients just by examining stool samples for characteristic changes in gut flora, without looking at any other clinical data. Long-haul symptoms are also strongly associated with characteristic changes in gut bacteria, like the ones just described in the study published in *Gut,* and there's lots of symptom overlap between the two conditions, especially persistent fatigue, brain fog, and muscle and joint aches.

There's no single test to confirm ME/CFS, and symptoms can mimic other health problems that cause extreme fatigue, including disorders like sleep apnea and insomnia, hypothyroidism, depression, and anxiety. It's common for people with ME/CFS to also have other health problems at the same time, like irritable bowel syndrome, fibromyalgia, and mood disorders, and that's also true of many people with long COVID.

Like other post-viral syndromes, treatment of ME/CFS focuses on symptom relief, and that includes treating any accompanying depression, pain, or sleep problems with counseling, diet, lifestyle interventions, and medication when appropriate. As evidence mounts that disruptions in gut flora are associated with conditions like ME/CFS, attention to rehabbing the microbiome through diet and lifestyle changes will likely start to play a bigger role in treatment.

POST-INFECTIOUS IBS

Post-infectious irritable bowel syndrome (PI-IBS) is a constellation of signs and symptoms that can develop after infection in the gut, and the condition has some similarities to what millions of people are now experiencing after they recover from the acute aspects of SARS-CoV-2 infection.

Symptoms of PI-IBS begin after an episode of acute gastroenteritis, and published studies report an incidence of between 5 percent and 32 percent after infection. A recent systematic review described a six-fold increased risk of IBS after infection, and that risk remains elevated for at least two to three years. Underlying mechanisms include persistent subclinical inflammation, disruption of intestinal barrier function leading to changes in intestinal permeability, and alteration of gut flora—all processes that are also at play with long COVID and other post-viral syndromes. People with underlying psychological disorders and those with severe initial gastroenteritis are most at risk.

One important point when dealing with PI-IBS is avoidance of antibiotics. When people return from an overseas trip with diarrhea, abdominal pain, nausea, and fatigue, their physician's first instinct is sometimes to treat them with strong antibiotics due to the possibility of a bacterial infection. As you can imagine, that only worsens any microbiome abnormalities that may have been present before the acute gastroenteritis or changes in gut flora that may have been caused by the infection—as we've seen with SARS-CoV-2. Because I practice in Washington, D.C., where there's a large international community, the State Department, the Peace Corps, and multiple embassies, I see lots of patients with PI-IBS. Most have gradual resolution of their symptoms without any intervention, but my microbiome rehab program for addressing dysbiosis outlined in the Anti-Viral Gut Plan speeds up that process and significantly decreases the likelihood they'll end up with chronic symptoms.

THE POST-VIRAL GUT-BRAIN CONNECTION

Some of the most troubling post-viral symptoms are invisible to the eye. Brain fog is a collection of neurological symptoms that can affect virus sufferers during and/or after their initial infection. It includes an inability to concentrate, absentmindedness, difficulty recalling or retaining information, fatigue, and changes in mood. As for a lot of other post-viral symptoms, there's no test to measure brain fog, and it's not yet really considered an official medical diagnosis. Brain fog has also been diagnosed in people who, to their knowledge, were never infected with a virus, maybe as a result of stress due to the pandemic. Constant broadcasts about the number of people dying, new variants that may be vaccine resistant, and other messaging that instills fear (and keeps us watching the news) cause a fight-or-flight stress response in the brain and the body that can lead to brain fog regardless of whether you've been infected or not.

We now know that many of these viral illnesses, including COVID, don't involve just the respiratory system but are actually systemic diseases that can affect many critical organs, including the brain. Neurological complications such as brain fog, confusion, dizziness, panic attacks, and even cognitive impairment resembling dementia are all part of the symptom complex of post-viral illnesses. Ironically, some of the medications prescribed for neuropsychiatric problems can actually increase the risk of dementia following COVID infection. A study published in March 2022 in *Frontiers in Medicine* revealed that antidepressants, benzodiazepines prescribed for stress and anxiety, mood stabilizers, and antipsychotics can all increase the risk of dementia after COVID. People over sixty-five taking these medications were up to three times more likely to develop dementia following a SARS-CoV-2 infection, and the risk is likely increased in younger people, too.

While some viruses can directly impact the brain, many post-viral neurological symptoms are multifactorial in origin. Medications that affect the brain are an important consideration, and so are behaviors that impact brain health. One of the most effective ways to resolve symptoms is therefore to examine behaviors that are associated with a lower likelihood of those symptoms developing. A study presented at the American Heart Association's Epidemiology, Prevention, Lifestyle and Cardiometabolic Health Scientific Sessions helps highlight some of these interventions. The study included 302,239 individuals aged fifty to seventy-three years with no dementia at baseline. Each participant completed baseline examinations from 2006 to 2010 as part of the UK Biobank study. Participants were categorized into groups based on the number of healthy behaviors they had from the following list:

1. BMI of less than 30 kg/m^2
2. Moderate to vigorous physical activity of at least 150 minutes per week
3. Sleep duration of six to nine hours per day
4. Drinking in moderation (0 to 14 drinks per week for men and 0 to 7 drinks per week for women)
5. Not smoking
6. Eating a healthy diet of more fruits and vegetables and fewer processed meats and refined grains

The study found that people who regularly engaged in three or more of the healthy behaviors had a significantly lower dementia risk, and that was true even for people at high risk due to familial dementia. The results provide important evidence that a healthy lifestyle can have a positive impact not just on physical health but on brain health, too, and gives us a clear guide to exactly what those behaviors are that greatly reduce the likelihood of cognitive decline. The range of behaviors speaks to the multifactorial nature of dementia. We can't draw a straight line from one specific behavior to the development (or improvement) of dementia or brain fog, and that's why it's important to pursue solutions that address all of these possible etiologies.

The best way to prevent post-viral symptoms is to not get infected with a virus, but for those who do, the best way to prevent neurological complications is to have a healthy brain at baseline. And the same is true for more general complications of viruses, which are best avoided by having a healthy gut at baseline. While it's not a guarantee, it's reassuring to know that consistently following a few healthy behaviors (and paying attention to what's in your medicine cabinet) can preserve your health and decrease the likelihood of chronic symptoms after viral illness.

TAKING ACTION

Chronic symptoms after COVID might be driven by the direct effects of the virus, but the additional indirect effects of reduced social contact, loneliness, incomplete recovery of physical health, loss of employment, and disordered sleep can also wreak havoc on your physical and emotional health. If you're struggling with post-viral symptoms, it doesn't matter whether you were in the ICU, mildly infected, or not sure whether you were infected at all; the trauma, the symptoms, and the suffering are real, and the solutions you'll find in the third part of this book will be helpful regardless of what category you fall into. Best of all, the recommendations for how to prevent infection or restore function after a viral illness are all research-backed health boosters with literally no downside. Let's get started!

To view the scientific references cited in this chapter, please visit
drrobynnechutkan.com/anti-viral-gut-references.

STRENGTHENING

PART 3

FROM WITHIN
THE ANTI-VIRAL GUT PLAN

I've provided you with a lot of scientific and clinical data about susceptibility to viruses in the first two parts of this book. Now let's focus on the specific steps that can protect you from current and future viral threats.

The first step is recognizing that it's not actually you that you're fortifying; it's your army of microbes. If you don't have a healthy population of virus-busting superstars like *Faecalibacterium prausnitzii*, and the ability to keep bandits like *Enterococcus faecalis* in check, the battle may be lost before it even begins.

The second step is understanding that you are actually preparing for battle. This isn't about detoxing, cleansing, or fitting into your skinny jeans. This is about surviving and thriving during one of the most dangerous periods in the last hundred years of human history. Be open to doing things differently and maybe even being a little inconvenienced.

The third and most important step is believing that you have some control over the outcome. Exposure to viruses does not have to lead to infection; infection does not have to lead to illness; and illness does not have to progress to death or debility. But that belief needs to be accompanied by action. Continuing to do what you've always done and simply hoping for the best is not enough. Neither is eating a suboptimal diet and taking a bunch of supplements that claim to boost your immune system.

If you're trying to win the war against viruses, your efforts need to be both external and internal: follow public health guidelines to limit your exposure to the virus *and* also do the internal work to strengthen your terrain. Remember, it's not just the potency of the pathogen that determines outcome; the health of the host is even more important! Multiple scientific studies confirm that your microbiome is *the* most accurate predictor of outcome—not just whether you'll recover from acute infection, but also your likelihood of developing prolonged symptoms. Creating a powerful anti-viral gut is not complicated, but it requires habit change and consistency, both of which can be challenging to embrace. While you don't have to adopt all the recommendations I'm going to be providing in the upcoming chapters, keep in mind that the more you do, the better your results.

REMOVE, REPLACE, RESTORE

The cornerstone of the Anti-Viral Gut Plan is three-pronged: *removing* medications, practices, and foods that are damaging to your microbiome; *replacing* missing or depleted essential bacteria through exposure to soil microbes, ferments, and robust pre-, pro-, and postbiotics; and *restoring* your gut shield with medicinal foods, select micronutrients, the right environment, and scientifically backed mind-body practices. The good news is you don't have to become a vegan or go all the way back to the cave to rewild yourself, although my Anti-Viral Gut Plan will show you how to bring some important elements of plant-based eating and cave life back home. If you suffer from dysbiosis, autoimmune disease, or other comorbidities, take medications that put you at risk, struggle with your weight, feel overwhelmed by stress, or simply want to safeguard against future viral illness, this plan will provide you with everything you need: what to eat and drink, lifestyle and mental health tactics, important tips to help strengthen host defenses, how to approach the medicine cabinet, a guide to probiotics and supplements, plus recipes to rehab your microbiome. Here's a preview of what you can expect:

Chapter 8: Building Up Your Body

A whole new way of looking at food and drink that emphasizes the blockbuster nutrients you need to grow a good gut garden. The plan is easy to adhere to because there's no calorie counting, and the focus is on what you're missing and need to add in rather than on what you should eliminate. Plus how much exercise and what type of workout should you be doing to boost your virus-fighting capabilities, and can exercise improve resiliency even if you're overweight?

Chapter 9: Securing Defenses

Host defenses are there to protect you—but only if you don't inadvertently dismantle them. Discover how to optimize your body's own innate capacity to neutralize, trap, burn, and wall off viruses, while simultaneously improving reflux symptoms, digestion, overall gut health, and your immune response.

Chapter 10: Mastering Your Mind

What you think is in your head is also in your body. Stress and sleep deprivation profoundly affect your gut and its army of microbes. Learn how to dial in simple solutions for relieving stress, getting a good night's sleep, and changing the negative chatter in your head to up your body's mental as well as physical resilience to viruses.

Chapter 11: Changing Your Environment

The Japanese practice of *shinrin yoku*, or "forest bathing," reduces stress hormone production, enhances your immune system, and accelerates recovery from illness. When combined with the anti-viral effects of open air, nature is powerful medicine. Just as adding in a healthy dose of nature improves your anti-viral response, toxic products can mess with your microbiome. Learn which products are the key offenders.

Chapter 12: Being Thoughtful About Therapeutics

Tackling health challenges without destroying precious microbes in the process involves knowing the critical questions to ask your doctor when you're sick, understanding how to protect your microbes when you're taking an antibiotic, being aware of which medications are detrimental to essential bacteria and should be avoided, plus having a comprehensive guide to probiotics and supplements that can make a difference when dealing with viruses.

Chapter 13: Plan at a Glance

Now that you know what to do, let's put it all together with a snapshot glance at what your daily anti-viral gut routine should look like.

Chapter 14: Recipes

Simple, delicious food to nourish you and your gut microbes.

Many of us have become alienated from our body's capacity to battle pathogens and believe pharmaceuticals and medical interventions are the only route to staying well. Medical care can play an important role, but there is no pill, potion, or device as powerful as your body's own ability to resist and recover from viral infections. Those abilities emanate from your gut, and optimizing them will provide you with the greatest degree of protection against viruses. Hippocrates said that *all disease begins in the gut*. Most solutions are to be found there, too. Whether you're trying to prevent infection, recovering from a recent viral illness, or dealing with chronic post-viral symptoms, the recommendations in this plan will help.

You can't control what's going on in the world, but you can control what's going on in the inner world of your terrain. Let's get started!

Building Up Your Body

FACT: What you eat has a bigger impact on your microbiome and its ability to protect you from viruses than anything else you do. The good news is microbial health is based on the sum total of what you eat, not on any one ingredient or food group. Gut bacteria need specific essential raw materials and nutrients to survive, and those requirements come from lots of different foods, which means you can eat a broad and bountiful diet while nourishing your microbes. The focus should be on adding the right stuff to your plate instead of worrying too much about what you need to eliminate, because it's the absence of beneficial fiber rather than the presence of the not-so-good foods that leads to a depleted microbiome. For most of us, eating enough lentils and leeks can balance out a slice of cake here and there. By adding in more of the raw materials your microbes rely on, you'll end up crowding out the less helpful foods, even if you don't eliminate them altogether. I'll point out what some of those less helpful foods are, as well as a few that can do real damage to your microbiome that you should definitely avoid.

FEED YOUR MICROBES

Let's start with some basic guidelines for what you should be feeding yourself—and your microbes—and then we'll get into the nitty-gritty of specific foods.

Eat More Plants

Plants, defined as vegetables, fruits, legumes, grains, nuts, and seeds (anything that comes out of the ground or off a shrub, vine, or tree), provide the raw material for bacterial fermentation, which produces short-chain fatty acids (SCFAs)—arguably the most important metabolites for gut and immune function, so eating more plants is the number one strategy for improving your gut shield. The diversity and number of plants you eat is reflected in the diversity and number of bacteria you grow in your gut, so you should try to eat lots of different types every day.

How do we know this? In 2018 researchers from the American Gut Project published the largest human microbiome study ever done, involving over ten thousand people from forty-five different countries. Their study confirmed that the number of plant types in your diet is the primary factor that determines the health and diversity of your gut microbiome. Regardless of what diet they ate (vegetarian, vegan, omnivore, etc.), participants who ate more than thirty different plant types per week had gut microbiomes that were much healthier than those who ate ten or fewer types of plants per week. This isn't just a theoretical improvement—the diversity in your microbiome cultivated by eating a wide variety of fibrous plants is directly correlated with better outcomes from viral infections.

But here's the problem: a report from the National Cancer Institute on the status of the American diet found that three out of four Americans don't eat a single piece of fruit in a given day, and nine out of ten don't reach the minimum recommended daily intake of vegetables. On a weekly basis, less than 5 percent of Americans achieve the minimum three servings a week for greens or beans, only 2 percent reach the minimum two servings a week for orange vegetables, and only 1 percent consume the recommended three to four ounces a day of whole grains. Almost the entire country is eating in a way that is virtually guaranteed to make them more susceptible to viruses and puts them at risk for poorer outcomes. Those habits are reflected in the tragically high rates at which the coronavirus has killed Americans.

But it doesn't have to be this way. We can fight viruses effectively and efficiently by changing what we feed ourselves—and our army of microbes. Focusing on getting more plants on your plate is the best way to start. A helpful way to think about the relationship between eating plants and gut bacteria is that the plant fiber that can't be broken down and absorbed by your body ends up feeding your bacteria instead. The tough fibrous part of plants, like the stems of broccoli or the base of asparagus, provide the most indigestible fiber, so make sure you're eating those parts, too.

My 1-2-3 rule can help you get more plant foods onto your plate every day. Here's how it works: eat one vegetable in the morning, two at lunch, and three at dinner. There are lots of ways to accomplish this. You could have a smoothie with kale or a spinach omelet for breakfast, salad with chopped raw veggies for lunch, and steamed asparagus plus a salad of lettuce and cucumbers with your dinner (or do what I do and make it 3-2-1 instead by starting off the morning with a green smoothie with at least three different vegetables in it). The 1-2-3 rule is a great way to make sure you're getting enough dietary fiber without getting bogged down in too many details and focusing on building your meal around plants will help you think about meat as a side dish rather than the main event—a great microbe-boosting strategy. Here are some additional tips for increasing the amount of plant fiber you're eating:

SUBSTITUTE
- zucchini "noodles" for wheat pasta
- roasted squash or sweet potato for french fries
- mashed green bananas for mashed potatoes
- mashed cauliflower for white rice

ADD IN

- spinach and kale to smoothies
- leeks and celery to soups and stews
- roasted pumpkin or squash instead of flour to thicken sauces
- onions, garlic, peppers, and spinach to scrambled eggs

PLANTS, NOT PILLS OR POWDERS

Getting your nutrients from food instead of through a pill or powder is always preferable because you get the entire spectrum of health-promoting ingredients when you eat the whole food instead of just one isolated ingredient that's often accompanied by undesirable fillers and binders. A good example are polyphenols, micronutrients that naturally occur in plants. They're touted in many supplements, but they're also super easy to get in your diet from foods like fruits, vegetables, teas, and spices, and of course eating those foods confers additional benefits beyond just supplying polyphenols. Green powders that claim to be the equivalent of eating vegetables are particularly problematic, since most vegetables start to wilt and lose their nutrient value shortly after harvesting. The idea that important nutrients in these foods can still be active several months after they're extracted just isn't plausible—or proven.

Choose Your Carbs Carefully

Many of us have been conditioned to think of carbohydrates as "bad" foods that make us fat and cause diabetes. But all carbs are definitely not created equal, and it's important to know which ones are actually good for your microbes and which ones you should avoid. Simple carbohydrates ("bad" carbs) found in soda, baked goods, and other processed foods are rapidly digested in your small intestine and absorbed as glucose. When you eat them, they cause a spike in your insulin levels and are associated with weight gain, diabetes, and in-flammation. They also cause unhealthy shifts in the composition of your microbiome and can lead to overgrowth of undesirable yeast species.

Complex carbohydrates ("good" carbs) are typically high in fiber and include foods like fruits, vegetables, some whole grains, beans, and brown rice. Because of their high fiber content, these foods don't cause a surge in insulin levels and, from a microbial point of view, they're some of the most important foods for nurturing essential microbes. Resistant starches and inulin are two types of good carbs that you need to know about, because they're great for your microbiome.

Resistant starches are a specific type of complex carbohydrate that don't get digested in your small intestine. They travel through your gastrointestinal (GI) tract relatively intact until they reach your colon, where they're fermented by gut bacteria to produce SCFAs. Resistant starches function more like dietary fiber than starch, encouraging the growth of healthy microbes in your colon and acting as a prebiotic food: one that actually feeds your gut bacteria and reduces production of potentially harmful compounds.

FOOD HIGH IN RESISTANT STARCHES
Green bananas
Green peas
Lentils
Uncooked rolled oats
White beans

Inulin is another type of complex carbohydrate known as a fructan. Like resistant starches, inulin also has prebiotic qualities: it feeds your microbes to promote healthy gut flora. Adding inulin-containing foods such as leeks to soups or stews, bananas to your green smoothies, and garlic and onion for sautéing whatever you're cooking can help to increase the amount of inulin in your diet.

FOODS HIGH IN INULIN
Artichokes
Asparagus
Bananas
Chicory root
Dandelion root
Garlic
Leeks
Onions

Ferment Your Food
Fermented vegetables such as sauerkraut, kimchi, and pickles are microbiome rock stars because they contain live bacteria (probiotics) *and* prebiotic fiber to nourish your gut bacteria. During the fermentation process the microorganisms in fermented foods produce lots of different nutrients, so a jar of sauerkraut is really a living food with vitamins and other helpful substances that are actively being produced. When you eat those foods, you're consuming all of those microbially produced substances that are good for you. A study by researchers at Stanford University published in the journal *Cell* found that eating fermented foods every day resulted in marked reductions in over a dozen different inflammatory compounds in the body, plus more diversity of gut bacteria. The more fermented foods people ate, the greater the number of microbial species that bloomed in their guts. These foods also activate antioxidants in humans, and they've been clinically proven to help reduce severity of viral illnesses like COVID.

You should try to include some fermented vegetables in your diet every day. They're super easy to make—mostly involving just adding a little sea salt and some water to veggies—and after fermenting, they can keep in your refrigerator for weeks. Check out Chapter 14, "Recipes," for some tasty examples. Unfortunately, fermented non-vegetable food and drink like yogurt and kombucha don't have the same benefits—I'll explain more below.

Eat Dirty Food

The main difference between the produce you buy at the supermarket and what you find at most farm stands is dirt and distance. These days, our produce travels long distances—sometimes thousands of miles from other continents—before it gets to us. The enzymatic activity and nutrient value of these foods starts to decline right after harvesting, and so does its microbial value. Buying locally grown food from small farmers means that the food has traveled a shorter distance to get to you, so more of the nutrients and bacteria are intact. You'll probably find that it stays fresh longer, too.

Chances are also higher that it's been grown in small batches in soil, rather than in the aseptic factory environment of mass-produced food. Look for produce that has evidence of dirt on it (although you still need to wash it before you eat it) and isn't perfectly uniform in color or size, reflecting the normal variation of food grown in nature, rather than engineered to look a certain way. And of course, organically produced food, grown with dirt rather than chemicals, is always best.

Farm Yes, Factory No

If you're ever in a bind about whether something is good for you or your microbes, this is my absolute favorite and simplest way to figure it out: If it came straight from the farm, go ahead. If it made a stop in a factory, don't bother. That means yes to apples but no to applesauce; yes to lentils but no to lentil chips; yes to brown rice but no to brown rice cereal. You get the gist.

. . . . .

Now that you're clear on what you should be emphasizing, let me tell you about some foods you might want to think about cutting back on, and some you should completely eliminate because they're actually hazardous to your gut health.

Manage Your Meat Intake

Remember the Italian researcher Paolo Lionetti who compared children eating a fiber-rich, plant-based diet with those eating a lot of sugar, fat, and animal protein? The results showed huge differences in gut bacteria: the high-animal-protein group had less microbial diversity and more species associated with illness, while the high-fiber group had higher levels of beneficial SCFAs and more health-promoting and virus-fighting species. But here's the bottom line: meat isn't necessarily bad for your microbiome, but dietary fiber is really good for it and eating too much of the former can lead to not eating enough of the latter. There's only so much room on your plate, and it's really important to make sure that the microbe-boosting foods are well represented. So ideally, you should think of the veggies as the main course and meat as a side dish (or skip it altogether). Make sure you're eating the best-quality, grass-fed meat available, with no antibiotics, since cows raised on corn or treated with antibiotics produce more pathogenic bacteria, such as *E. coli* O157:H7, that can disrupt your microbiome and make you more susceptible to viral infections.

Cut Back on Sugar

Sugar feeds gut bacteria—but not the kind you're trying to encourage. A diet high in sugar can lead to overgrowth of yeast species and pathogenic bacteria. It can also compromise your ability to fight viruses by interfering with your white blood cells' ability to destroy pathogens—and that effect starts within minutes of eating sugar and can last for several hours. So, in addition to causing imbalance in your microbiome, sugar can actually impair your body's ability to fight viruses.

What makes it all so hard to give up is that sugar is habit-forming: it increases the microbial populations that thrive on it, which then increase your cravings for more sugar, and it also activates opiate receptors in your brain, which gives you a pleasurable "sugar high" when you eat it. I recommend cutting down on sugar gradually: decrease the amount of sweetener you're using; eat fewer processed and packaged foods since they tend to have a lot of added sugar; get rid of candy, soda, and sweetened drinks, which almost always contain high fructose corn syrup—one of the most unhealthy sweeteners; and satisfy your cravings with dark chocolate (70 percent cacao or higher) and fruit instead. Whether you gradually reduce your sugar consumption or do a more drastic sugar detox, your gut bacteria should eventually get to the point where the sugar-craving microbes are outnumbered and your cravings become easier to control.

Can't give it up completely? Honey has a lower glycemic index than regular sugar, which means it releases less glucose into your bloodstream, and in some studies it has been described as having prebiotic properties, so it's a reasonable alternative to sugar (although if you suffer from severe forms of dysbiosis, including yeast overgrowth, you may want to use honey more sparingly). High-nutrient raw versions such as manuka honey are what I recommend. Agave is a natural sweetener but, as with honey, too much can still be a problem, so they both fall into the "one serving a day" category. Stevia has been marketed as a healthy low-calorie sweetener, but studies show that, like other artificial sweeteners, it's also disruptive to gut microbes so should be avoided. If you're finding it hard to give up dessert, here are some ways you can still enjoy a sweet treat while reducing your sugar intake:

- frozen bananas blended with almond butter "ice cream"
- dates filled with nut butter
- raw honey instead of sugar when baking, and halve the amount called for in the recipe
- fresh ginger instead of sugar in herbal tea or lemonade

Be Thoughtful About Dairy

An astounding 80 percent of all antibiotics sold in the United States are used in the food industry—primarily to treat infections or to promote faster growth in animals raised for human consumption. The Food and Drug Administration (FDA) requires that milk contain no detectable antibiotics when tested, but random inspections have found dairy cows with illegal levels of antibiotics, raising concerns about their presence in the U.S. milk supply, which could be contributing to the rise of widespread antibiotic resistance in humans—and affecting our microbiome.

First developed by Louis Pasteur in 1864, pasteurization kills harmful organisms responsible for diseases like typhoid fever and tuberculosis and involves heating dairy products like milk to very high temperatures, then rapidly cooling them to decrease spoilage from bacteria and extend their shelf life. The problem with pasteurization is that it also destroys most of the naturally occurring helpful bacteria and vitamins in milk. Some alternative health practitioners recommend raw, unpasteurized dairy products as a source of beneficial bacteria, but those will still cause problems if you're lactose intolerant, like 70 percent of the world's population.

The purpose of cow's milk is to nurture calves, just like breast milk is incredibly important for our babies, but the clinical and scientific data for recommending dairy—including fermented products like yogurt and cheese that have been pasteurized—as a way to enhance the anti-viral capabilities of our own gut flora just isn't there. Enjoy dairy sparingly as a treat, but not as a health food with the ability to meaningfully improve your microbiome.

Eliminate Frankenfoods

Staying away from foods that have been modified and adulterated from what nature intended (like genetically modified organisms—GMOs) is good for your microbiome for a number of reasons: they may have additives and preservatives that can be harmful to gut bacteria, they may be full of hormones or may contain detectable levels of antibiotics, they may have been sprayed with pesticides that are toxic to your microbiome, our GI tracts may have a hard time digesting them, most of the healthy fiber may have been removed during processing, or they may not provide enough nutrients to encourage the growth of healthy bacteria. Refined carbohydrates like pastries and breakfast cereals, processed foods in general, genetically modified foods, and artificial sweeteners all fit the bill.

THE ANTI-VIRAL GUT DIET

Now that you're familiar with the general guidelines about what to emphasize and what to cut back on, let's profile the foods in your day-to-day diet in a little more detail. In line with my goal of keeping eating easy and pleasurable, I've divided the food lists below into three types: green-light foods, which you can eat as much as you like; yellow-light foods, which I recommend you limit to one serving a day; and red-light foods, which you should try to avoid.

Green-Light Foods

Most of these foods contain lots of plant fiber to nourish your microbes, others have healthy fats like omega-3 fatty acids that have anti-inflammatory properties, and some don't have specific microbe-boosting features but can be enjoyed without any ill effects on your gut bacteria. You can eat as many of these foods as you need to feel full—don't worry about calories or portion size because most of these foods have a very favorable nutrient-per-calorie index, meaning they deliver lots of nutrients to your body for each calorie consumed. Don't forget to include plenty of prebiotic foods such as onions, garlic, leeks, artichokes, beans, asparagus, carrots, radishes, as well as fermented foods such as sauerkraut and kimchi.

Fruits

Vegetables

Root vegetables

Nuts and nut butters

Seeds (including flaxseed)

Legumes (beans, peas, peanuts, chickpeas, lentils)

Olive oil

Coconut oil

Avocado oil

Sweet potato

White potato

Squash

Unprocessed gluten-free whole grains like brown rice, teff, etc.

Oats (steel-cut or old-fashioned)

Quinoa

Unsweetened dried fruits

Green-Light Baking
Almond flour
Coconut flour
Chickpea flour
Brown rice flour
Green banana flour

Yellow-Light Foods
These foods aren't specifically beneficial for your microbiome, but they can still be enjoyed in moderation. Limit your consumption to one serving daily. Organic, antibiotic-free animal products are best.
Wild-caught fish
Wild game
Grass-fed beef
Organic meat/poultry/eggs
Ghee/clarified butter
Organic raw honey or agave

Red-Light Foods
When consumed regularly, these foods are associated with dysbiosis, either because they're broken down into simple sugars upon digestion, are highly processed, or contain ingredients that damage the intestinal lining or the microbes that live there. Try to avoid these foods.
Dairy (except ghee/clarified butter)
Sugar
Artificial sweeteners (aspartame, stevia, sorbitol, mannitol, etc.)
High fructose corn syrup
Processed corn products (non-GMO corn on the cob is fine)
Gluten
Processed carbohydrates
Refined oils (canola, safflower, etc.)

When considering what to eat to create a strong anti-viral gut, re-member what I told you at the beginning of this section about the sum total being the most important factor. Don't fret or obsess over any single ingredient or item on any of the lists. Just try to eat as many things from the farm and as few from the factory as possible and you—and your microbes—will be fine.

Drink Up

Hydrating your body serves two specific anti-viral functions: it helps improve the barrier function of your skin and mucous membranes to keep viruses out, and it helps to flush toxins and pathogens out of your body. Your skin, digestive tract, and kidneys are your main organs of elimination, and they all rely on adequate amounts of fluid to do their job. Even mild dehydration can have a big impact on that—losing just 2 percent of your body's water can decrease skin elasticity and strength, slow down transit time in your gut, and put extra strain on your heart and kidneys. The reality is by the time most people feel thirsty, they're already dehydrated, so it's really important to monitor and maintain adequate fluid intake before that happens. And keep in mind that if you do get infected with a virus, symptoms like coughing, sneezing, fever, vomiting, and diarrhea all create dehydration and can prolong symptoms, so hydration is a big part of both prevention and recovery from viruses.

Brain fog after a viral illness often has multiple contributing causes, but improving it may involve some simple tactics, like drinking more water. Your brain is 75 percent water, and when you're dehydrated, it has a much more difficult time functioning. In young people, symp-toms of dehydration can be reversed by just replacing fluids. But as we get older, our brains become more vulnerable, and dehydration can lead to cognitive impairment, especially if there was already some pre-existing decline. Brain fog and cognitive impairment aren't single entities; they're complex conditions with multiple different factors that contribute to their development. If you have post-viral symptoms and risk factors for neurological dysfunction, including diabetes, obesity, cardiovascular disease, hypertension, or a nutrient deficient diet, and you're also dealing with dehydration on a regular basis, the fluid loss can tip you over the edge and create an opportunity for brain fog and impairment to set in. It's like being sleep-deprived and physically exhausted, taking medication that makes you drowsy, having a few beers, and then deciding to take a drive. Any one of those things on their own might be manageable, but the combination can be deadly when you get behind the wheel of a car.

If you're over sixty and dealing with post-viral symptoms, especially if you're female, you need to be particularly attuned to your water intake. Women are more sensitive to the neurological effects of dehydration because they have a higher percentage of fat tissue than men, which has a lower water composition compared to lean tissue. Older women are especially vulnerable: a study examining the hydration status of adults over age sixty found that dehydrated women performed much worse on tasks related to attention and processing speed, and significantly worse than men who were dehydrated.

So how much water do you need to make sure you're adequately hydrated? You may feel like you're already drinking a lot, but current hydration recommendations are actually more than they have been in the past. The National Academy of Medicine recommends that in order to stay adequately hydrated, men should drink about 125 ounces of water daily and woman should drink about 90, but a solid rule of thumb is to drink at least half your body weight in ounces of water. Make sure you're drinking enough to result in frequent clear urination. (If your pee is yellow, you're definitely still dehydrated.) And despite all the marketing around sports drinks, rehydration solutions, and electrolyte replenishers, plain old water is still the best way to hydrate yourself. Here are a couple of additional options for fluids that won't disrupt your microbes or the rest of your body:

Green-Light Drinks
Water
Carbonated water
Unsweetened, unflavored coconut water
Dairy substitutes: almond milk, hemp milk, cashew milk, coconut milk (unsweetened and with no additives)
Herbal tea
Smoothies
Vegetable juices (with no added sugar or sweeteners)

And here are some that you should have a little less of (one serving daily), or avoid, because the ingredients (excess chemicals and sugar) are problematic for your gut flora:

Yellow-Light Drinks
Alcohol
Kombucha
Coffee

Red-Light Drinks
Sodas
Diet sodas
Fruit juices

Some of us can tolerate a little alcohol without any serious health repercussions, but there are categories of people who should definitely avoid it altogether. Studies show that just one drink per day in women and two in men can induce dysbiosis, damage your liver, increase the permeability of your gut, and affect your immune system. When you're exposed to a virus, your body mounts an immune response to attack and kill it. In general, the healthier your immune system, the quicker it can clear the virus and the faster you can recover. Alcohol makes it harder for your immune system to do its job defending you against pathogens. In the lungs, alcohol damages immune cells that are responsible for clearing the virus out of your airway. In the gut, it triggers inflammation and destroys microorganisms that maintain immune health, leading to an increased risk of infections and complications. If you're at high risk for viral infections (older, immunocompromised, obese, have autoimmune disease or diabetes) or trying to recover from post-viral symptoms, abstinence is definitely the way to go. It doesn't make sense to ingest a known toxin on a regular basis while you're trying to restore your health.

Kombucha has been touted as a health aid, but its microbial benefits haven't been proven, and some brands contain a lot of sugar. To make kombucha, strains of bacteria, yeast, and sugar are added to tea and fermented at room temperature, which produces bacteria and yeast known as a SCOBY (symbiotic culture of bacteria and yeast). While many in the beverage industry hype the benefits of these live bacteria as having helpful probiotic qualities, the bacteria from kombucha generally don't survive intact through your stomach to be able to colonize your colon. And while studies have shown that different brands of kombucha do indeed contain live beneficial bacteria, there's no compelling data to show that these bacteria actually improve the composition or diversity of your microbiome. Still, a glass of kombucha—especially one with low amounts of sugar and no artificial sweeteners—can be a better alternative to soda or alcohol when you have a taste for something other than water. Just don't rely on it as part of your anti-viral strategy.

Making sure you're well hydrated strengthens your defensive barriers, improves viral elimination routes, and can play a big role in preventing and recovering from post-viral symptoms like brain fog. Now would be a good time to pour yourself a tall glass of water and drink up!

GET MOVING

I don't need to tell you that exercise is good for you, but it turns out it's also really good for your gut microbes. A study published in the *British Journal of Sports Medicine* found that people who exercised at least five days a week had a 50 percent lower risk for upper respiratory viral infections and less severe symptoms when they were sick. Another British study compared stool samples from professional rugby players in the midst of their training season to those of healthy men of the same age who weren't avid exercisers. The athletes' stool samples had greater species diversity and significantly higher levels of beneficial species than their peers (not coincidentally, the rugby players also ate a lot more fruit and vegetables).

The good news is you don't need to be a professional rugby player or work out every day to benefit from the microbe-boosting effects of exercise. Just elevating your heart rate to 20 percent above baseline with a brisk walk for thirty minutes three to five times a week is enough to stimulate peristalsis, which keeps the products of digestion moving and increases your lymphatic flow, the fluid that surrounds your cells and transports metabolic waste—including viruses and other pathogens—out of your body.

Other ways exercise increases your immunity to viral illnesses include:

- Flushing pathogens out of your lungs and airways
- Increasing circulation of white blood cells and antibodies so they can detect illness earlier

- Elevating your body temperature, which helps you fight infection better
- Slowing down the release of stress hormones

When it comes to exercise, we've been taught that moderation is key to preventing injury and optimizing the immune benefits and that high-intensity exercise may actually depress your immune system as a result of increases in stress hormones. But there's now growing evidence that heavy exercise decreases your risk of upper respiratory tract infections through favorable changes in immune function without any negative effects of the stress hormones. That may be particularly true in people who find endurance activities like long-distance running to be stress-relieving rather than inciting. Regardless of how intensely you're working out, exercise is only a helpful anti-viral strategy if you're actually doing it regularly, and studies have shown that people are most likely to stick with more moderate exercise programs consisting of activities like:

- Cycling a few times a week
- Taking daily thirty- to sixty-minute walks or runs
- Doing strength training every other day
- Having a regular yoga practice

Like moving your body, giving your lungs a workout can have important health benefits, too, and regular use of a small and inexpensive breathing device called an incentive spirometer is an easy way to accomplish that. Ten deep breaths with it a couple of times a day keeps your lungs expanded and helps prevent both viral and bacterial pneumonia, which can develop when you're spending a lot of time sitting or lying on your back and not taking deep breaths. Both healthy people and those with lung disease can benefit from this type of pulmonary exercise to increase the capacity of their lungs, much the same way elite athletes do breathing exercises to increase their vital capacity so they can run more efficiently. A basic incentive spirometer costs less than $10 and, in addition to keeping your lungs in shape, will improve your overall cardiovascular fitness and exercise tolerance, too.

Just a reminder that if you're significantly overweight, regular exercise can decrease complications and death from viral infections, even without substantial weight loss. Exercise improves your terrain, so regardless of the number on the scale, it's still well worth the effort to try to work up a sweat.

Just like there aren't any bad vegetables, there aren't really any bad forms of exercise, although some can be more dangerous, inconvenient, or harder to master. Pick something that works for you and make it a regular part of your anti-viral routine.

Beyond food, drink, and exercise, there are some other important ways we can shore up our host defenses. Let's take a look at how preserving stomach acid, maximizing mucus, knowing when to let a fever run its course, and avoiding leaks in your gut can make you an even stronger adversary.

To view the scientific references cited in this chapter, please visit drrobynnechutkan.com/anti-viral-gut-references.

Securing Defenses

In earlier chapters, I mentioned important host defenses like stomach acid that inactivates viruses, mucus that traps and expels them, fever that brings viral replication to a standstill, and the gut epithelial barrier that keeps viruses out of your body. Now let's dive in to how to maintain—and even enhance—these critical weapons so they can do their job of keeping you safe from viruses.

MAINTAIN YOUR STOMACH ACID

Stomach acid is one of your main defenses against viruses. Luckily, when left to its own devices, your stomach makes plenty of it. The problem occurs when, in an attempt to alleviate symptoms like heartburn and acid reflux, you decide to block it with a proton pump inhibitor (PPI) and create an even bigger problem instead. PPIs transform your stomach into a friendly place for viruses to grow and multiply and are associated with an up-to-fourfold increased risk of viral illnesses like COVID. So what should you do if you suffer from acid reflux or heartburn and you want to treat your symptoms but still maintain your stomach acid? The guidelines below will help you keep symptoms under control so you can skip the acid suppression and make sure your stomach is well equipped to dismantle viruses.

- Give your stomach a curfew. The churning movements in your stomach that help propel food from north to south are tied to the circadian rhythm and slow to a standstill once the sun sets—which is ideally when you should stop eating.
- Calorie shift. Eat your largest meal early in the day when your stomach is most active and your smallest meal at night: breakfast like a king/queen, lunch like a prince/princess, and dinner like a pauper.
- Don't skip meals. That usually results in overeating later at night when your stomach is much less active—and that means more chances for food to reflux back up into your esophagus.
- Eat out early. If you're going to eat out, make it lunch or brunch rather than dinner.
- Eat small, frequent meals (especially for your meals later in the day). Your stomach is about the size of your fist. It can be stretched to a much larger capacity, but this will usually cause reflux symptoms. Eating mini-meals every three to four hours will keep you from getting hungry while also giving your stomach enough time to empty in between meals.
- Split servings. Consider taking your usual meal and splitting it into two servings a few hours apart to avoid overfilling your stomach.
- Wait four hours after eating to exercise or lie down so gravity can help your stomach empty while you're upright.
- Go for a walk after meals. Movement encourages peristalsis and will help speed up stomach emptying and prevent reflux.
- Watch out for fatty foods. Limit your consumption of foods with a high fat content that slow down stomach emptying, such as meat, cheese, and cream sauces.
- Cut down on dairy, caffeine, and alcohol. Dairy has a naturally high fat content, which can slow down stomach emptying

and cause reflux. Caffeine can cause the valve between your esophagus and stomach to open appropriately, and alcohol can also exacerbate reflux symptoms.

- Split up your fiber consumption. Definitely continue to eat lots of fiber, but if you're prone to reflux symptoms you may need to avoid eating a large amount of fiber at one sitting, which can lead to a full stomach and reflux.

- Sip, don't gulp. Hydration is important for keeping the products of digestion moving, but chugging on large amounts of fluid can precipitate reflux symptoms. Sip on fluids throughout the day instead, and drink liquids in between rather than during meals to avoid overfilling your stomach.

- Raise the head of your bed. Elevating the head of your bed a few inches may help to relieve nighttime reflux symptoms by providing a little help from gravity to keep stomach contents from refluxing back up.

Tapering PPIs

So let's say you follow all my diet and lifestyle tips above, and your acid reflux improves, but you're still taking a PPI every day and you'd like to discontinue it. Be sure to check with your health care provider first, but here's some important information about how to safely and effectively taper off.

The first thing to keep in mind is that these drugs are potent acid suppressors, so when you stop taking them, there may be a surge of acid that can make your reflux symptoms even worse. As acid levels begin to normalize, you'll start to feel better, but this can take several weeks, and many people don't make it through this challenging period and end up restarting their PPI. In order to get off them successfully, you'll need to be as strict as possible with your diet while you're tapering. Once you're off the drug for a few weeks, you can start to slowly reintroduce some of what you're missing to see how you tolerate it—but pay attention to any feedback your body gives you as you start to liberalize your diet. The goal isn't to keep you in food jail perpetually, it's to see what can be reincorporated safely and what you may need to continue to avoid in order to feel well. Follow my tips above to increase your chances of success. Here's a recommended six-week taper schedule for PPIs that's designed to minimize the acid surge:

Take one pill every other day for weeks one and two, then one pill every third day for weeks three and four, then one pill once a week for weeks five and six, and then stop taking the medication altogether.

Note: You can use shorter-acting antacids like Tums or H2 blockers like famotidine once or twice daily as needed while tapering and once you're off your PPI for good. And remember to check with your doctor first before discontinuing PPIs or any prescription medication.

Producing acid is a very natural and important part of what your stomach does. While there's some variation with how much stomach acid different people make, overproduction of acid is really uncommon, and so is underproduction. There's a slight decrease in levels as we age, but the overwhelming majority of people have sufficient amounts of stomach acid to denature viruses—unless they're on a proton pump inhibitor. In the absence of rare conditions like pernicious anemia and certain types of gastric bypass weight loss surgery, there's no indication to try to "acidify" your stomach either with an acid supplement or by drinking apple cider vinegar. Just let your stomach do what it does best, and you'll have plenty of acid to help keep you safe from viruses.

KEEP YOUR MUCUS MOIST AND HEALTHY

You may not think much about what's involved with maintaining healthy mucus production, active cilia, and an intact cough reflex—

until they go awry. But these critical host defenses can be sabotaged pretty easily—mostly by taking medications that suppress them and put you at risk for viral infections. Here are some ideas for relieving symptoms without compromising your amazing, lubricating, virus-trapping mucus.

HYDRATE: To keep mucus healthy and the right consistency, make sure you're well hydrated, especially in the winter. That means drinking at least 125 ounces of water for men and 90 ounces for women. At a bare minimum, you should be getting 8 cups a day—anything less puts you at risk for dried-out, cracked mucus membranes that will make you more vulnerable to viral penetration.

HUMIDIFY: Keep the air moist with a humidifier in your bedroom, which can help prevent your mucus membranes from becoming dried out. It doesn't matter whether you get a hot or cold air humidifier, but make sure you clean it regularly to avoid bacterial contamination.

FILTER: Use filters on your cooling and heating systems, and make sure you change them on a regular schedule.

RINSE: Consider using a neti pot—a container designed to rinse debris or excess mucus from your nasal cavity. If you decide to make your own saltwater solution, use distilled or sterilized bottled water. If you use a store-bought solution or nasal spray, make sure the ingredients are just salt and water and no additional chemicals.

AERATE: Invest in an incentive spirometer, a simple device that costs less than $10. It helps train you how to take deep breaths that can help air out your lungs and improve your cough reflex.

STEAM: Introduce warm moist air into your airways and sinus passages by sitting in a steam room or steam shower, or by putting your face over a bowl of steaming hot water and covering it with a towel (be careful not to burn yourself!). You can also wrap a hot towel around your face, but again, check the temperature first.

OIL: Eucalyptus oil acts on receptors in your nasal mucus membranes and can help reduce stuffiness. Use a few drops in your steam inhalation or on your hot towel, but avoid direct contact with your skin or internal surfaces.

SOOTHE: There's no compelling scientific evidence to suggest that the herbal remedy echinacea—a flowering plant in the daisy family commonly called coneflowers—helps reduce the severity or length of a cold, but many people find lozenges or tea containing echinacea soothing.

RIDE OUT A FEVER

If fever helps fight viruses, is there ever a situation where you should take fever-reducing drugs like ibuprofen or acetaminophen (Tylenol) when you're sick? Whether it's safe to ride out a fever depends on your age, underlying health, and what's causing it. Although infection is the most common cause, inflammation, flare-ups of autoimmune diseases like Crohn's or rheumatoid arthritis, allergies, drug reactions, vaccines, heat exhaustion, and even some kinds of cancer can also increase your core temperature and cause a fever, and these are all conditions that warrant medical attention, so it's always a good idea to seek a doctor's advice if you're not sure.

Assessment

Fevers are generally more worrisome in infants and children than in adults, because their ability to balance heat loss and gain isn't as well developed, so it's reasonable to have a lower threshold for seeking medical advice for them. The first thing you need to do when you think your core temperature might be elevated is confirm if you really have a fever. Oral thermometers are the most reliable, although rectal thermometers should be used in infants. Tympanic (ear) or skin thermometers aren't recommended because they're often inaccurate. Once you've established that you or your child has a fever, you don't need to keep checking it over and over again, unless there are accompanying signs that are changing, too, like becoming more irritable or lethargic, or developing a stiff neck or light sensitivity. But again, it's not the fever that's the focus here—it's trying to figure out the underlying cause, and a progression of symptoms even with no progression of fever can be cause for concern.

Young Children
If your baby or young child has a fever but is responsive, alert, making eye contact with you, responding to your voice, drinking fluids, and playing, there's probably no reason to be worried, but here are some febrile scenarios that should trigger a call or visit with a medical professional:

• Less than three months old with a rectal temperature of 100.4ºF or higher
• Three to six months old with a rectal temperature up to 102ºF, plus seems unusually irritable, lethargic, or uncomfortable, or has a temperature higher than 102ºF
• Six to twenty-four months old with a rectal temperature higher than 102ºF that lasts longer than one day but with no other symptoms. If other signs and symptoms are present (cough, diarrhea, etc.), you might call sooner based on the severity of the symptoms
• A fever and is listless or irritable, vomits repeatedly, has a severe

headache or stomachache, or has any other symptoms causing significant discomfort

- A fever after being left in a hot car—seek medical care immediately
- A fever that lasts longer than three days
- A fever and appears listless and has poor eye contact with you
- A fever in a child with a compromised immune system or a serious preexisting illness

Adults and Older Children

A temperature of 103°F or higher, especially if accompanied by any of the following signs or symptoms, should prompt you to seek medical attention:

- Severe headache
- Unusual skin rash, especially if the rash worsens rapidly
- Sensitivity to bright light
- Stiff neck and pain when you bend your head forward
- Mental confusion
- Persistent vomiting
- Difficulty breathing or chest pain
- Abdominal pain or pain when urinating
- Convulsions or seizures
- A compromised immune system or a serious preexisting illness

Treatment

A fever can make you or your child feel pretty crummy. Although by now you're probably convinced that automatically reaching for a drug to normalize temperature isn't necessarily a good idea, you may still want to alleviate some of the symptoms that are making you uncomfortable. Here are a couple of basic things you can do that won't interfere with the virus-fighting process of your fever but will make you feel a lot better:

HYDRATE: If you have a fever plus extreme achiness, a pounding headache, or fatigue, hydrating with water may be all you need to start feeling better. Fever increases insensible water losses as your body loses heat through your skin in an attempt to control core temperatures, so dehydration almost always accompanies a fever. Make sure you're drinking enough water to result in frequent clear urination. (If your pee is yellow, you're definitely still dehydrated.) Think of 64 ounces as the bare minimum and work your way up from there. Your thirst mechanism doesn't kick in until you're severely dehydrated, and even then, it can be hard getting in enough water because fever also suppresses your appetite and makes you less thirsty. Skip the vitamin water, sports drinks, or other adulterated versions of the real thing. Those drinks often have chemicals and sweeteners in them that can cause stomach upset and diarrhea and aren't as good at hydrating you as regular water. If you absolutely must have something with a little flavor and sweetness, or you're sweating a lot, try coconut water, which is full of helpful electrolytes and readily available at most supermarkets, but make sure it's unflavored with no added ingredients. A little salty broth in addition to water is good for replenishing electrolytes, too.

REST: This should be fairly intuitive, and your fever will probably be forcing you to slow down anyway, but rest allows your body to devote more resources to the important work of healing damaged tissues and fighting pathogens. Sitting or lying down in a cool, dark room can feel soothing and encourage you to rest.

STAY COOL: Using a cold compress, sucking on a Popsicle, making the ambient temperature in the room cool (but not cold), wearing light pajamas or clothing, and avoiding heavy blankets if you have a chill will all help you avoid overheating and keep you cool. Sitting in a bath of lukewarm water or giving yourself a sponge bath can also help you feel cooler and naturally lower your core temperature by a degree or two.

WAIT IT OUT: If you ultimately do end up taking an antipyretic, waiting a few hours before you take it may provide enough time to boost your immune response if you're otherwise healthy.

AVOID LEAKS

There's no miracle antidote for a leaky gut (and beware of untested supplement "cures" that claim to be), but there are definitely things you can do to help heal inflammation and restore the integrity of your gut lining. These solutions focus on removing offending agents, adding in good bacteria in your gut, and repairing the damage to your intestinal lining.

- Avoid medications like nonsteroidal anti-inflammatory drugs (NSAIDs), aspirin, antibiotics, steroids, and other agents that can damage your intestinal lining.
- Incorporate an anti-inflammatory diet that eliminates/reduces refined sugars, dairy, gluten, alcohol, and artificial sweeteners—some of the biggest offenders when it comes to inflammation in the gut that can compromise your barrier function. The recommendations for what to eat (and avoid) in the Anti-Viral Gut Diet are exactly what you should be following if you're trying to mend a leaky gut.
- If you're trying to increase levels of short-chain fatty acids (SCFAs) to help maintain the integrity of your gut lining, you

can't just take a butyrate supplement and call it a day. You have to actually increase your consumption of the foods that these helpful SCFA-producing microbes eat. The simplest way to do that is to eat more plant fiber, which also happens to be the most effective therapy for a leaky gut. Refer to my food plan for lots of tips on how to fill up on green leafy vegetables and other high-fiber foods that promote the growth of good bacteria in your gut.

- Don't forget to also include some fermented products like sauerkraut and non-dairy kefir that increase your ratio of good to bad bacteria and help keep your gut epithelial barrier healthy and intact.

- Think about adding a robust probiotic with large amounts of health-promoting *Bifidobacterium* and *Lactobacillus* species. When used in conjunction with dietary change, these can help restore balance in your gut flora (see Chapter 12 for how to select a probiotic).

- Consume lots of anti-inflammatory essential omega-3 fatty acids in foods like fish, flax, hemp, wheat germ, and walnuts. They're a key part of an anti-inflammatory diet since your body can't make them on its own. I recommend getting most of your nutrients from real food rather than supplements, but if allergies or the mercury content in fish prevent you from getting enough omega-3s, you can take 600 to 1,000 milligrams of a fish-oil supplement containing the omega-3 fatty acid docosahexaenoic acid (DHA). If you prefer not to consume animal products, you can substitute flaxseed oil, chia seeds, and purslane, which contain the plant-based omega-3 alpha-linolenic acid (ALA) or take 600 to 1,000 milligrams of an ALA supplement.

- Glutamine is an amino acid that your cells use to make protein and as an energy source. Your intestinal lining cells are avid consumers of glutamine, which has been shown in a few studies to help with intestinal injury after chemotherapy and radiation and may be beneficial in leaky gut (and I emphasize the "may" here). Safe doses in human studies range from 5 grams to about 15 grams daily.

Remember, we're still learning about leaky gut, so these supplement recommendations are mostly drawn from small clinical trials and anecdotal observation and aren't based on rigorous scientific studies. They are, however, reasonable recommendations with a low risk of side effects that, when combined with dietary changes, could help improve your intestinal permeability.

Now let's transition from shoring up our host defenses to shoring up our inner well-being, to make sure we're well equipped to take on viruses.

To view the scientific references cited in this chapter, please visit drrobynnechutkan.com/anti-viral-gut-references.

Mastering Your Mind

Stomach acid, mucus, and an intact gut lining are all critically important in protecting you from viruses, but so are the factors that you can't see, like your state of mind and your sleep status. Let's explore some of these mind-based modalities that are every bit as powerful as their body-based counterparts.

DE-STRESS YOURSELF

In my first book, *Gutbliss*, I talked about the biofeedback practitioner Emily Perlman, who worked her relaxation magic part-time in my office. She helped my patients with serious autoimmune diseases like Crohn's and ulcerative colitis, as well as people dealing with esophageal spasm, constipation, bloating, and all sorts of other gastrointestinal (GI) problems by quieting their mind and getting their breath and heart rate into a peaceful sync. One of the dramatic things I noticed in those patients, in addition to their GI symptoms improving, is that they became much more resilient to getting sick. Coughs, colds, the flu, and viral gastroenteritis were all much less common when their stress response was optimized. Although we know that's how it works in theory, it was impressive to see it actually manifesting in my patients. I'm excited to share some of these same anti-viral mind-based practices with you in this chapter.

In order to improve your stress response, you need to understand what triggers it in the first place, so let's do a quick review. Your nervous system is divided up into a central nervous system (CNS) and peripheral nervous system (PNS). Your CNS consists of your brain and spinal cord. Your PNS encompasses all the nerves outside your brain and spinal cord and is divided into a somatic nervous system, which is responsible for voluntary actions like moving your arms and legs, and an autonomic nervous system (ANS), which controls involuntary responses like your heart rate, blood pressure, respiration, and digestion. Your ANS is the part of your nervous system that's most involved in your stress response. It's further divided into a sympathetic nervous system, which controls the fight-or-flight response that's active during a threat or perceived danger, and your parasympathetic nervous system, which restores your body to a state of calm. So to summarize: your sympathetic nervous system revs you up and your parasympathetic nervous system calms you down. The goal is to make sure that your parasympathetic pathway, which is leading you to a nice, relaxed state, is more active than your sympathetic, which is getting you hyped up to do battle or flee.

Stressful events result in activation of your fight-or-flight sympathetic system. And since stress can hugely compromise your immune system and make you more vulnerable to viruses, improving resiliency needs to include controlling stress and figuring out how to deactivate your sympathetic nervous system.

You Have the Power

For most people, chronic stress (the bad kind) is subconscious and not something you can voluntarily turn on or off. But what you can control is your response—you can mindfully and intentionally create a healthier way of reacting to stress. Most stress is situational, but different people respond differently to the same set of stressors. Even if you're the ultimate type A control freak who has a hard time letting go, you can train yourself—the same way you learn how to hit a tennis ball, ride a bike, or play the piano—to change your response to stressful circumstances, and with enough practice, you can get really good at it. Since our world is getting more chaotic—and more dangerous in terms of infectious threats—honing your "relaxation response" is a great investment and doesn't cost you anything except time and effort. I'll explain exactly what the relaxation response is later in this section and give you specific advice on how to achieve it.

Although some people just seem to be born more relaxed and chill than others, feeling stressed and anxious are primarily learned behaviors. They're ways of looking at the world and responding to stimuli that are absorbed and emulated based on the people and the circumstances around you, and they can be unlearned, or at least redirected. Even if you've always been an anxious person or come from a really stressed-out, nervous family, you can break the cycle. Just like feeding yourself nourishing food, making sure you're adequately hydrated, and getting regular exercise, optimizing your stress response is a small act that produces big results. A healthy stress response yields a healthy immune response, which yields a healthy anti-viral response. It's all connected!

General Principles of De-stressing

Here are some guidelines for how to approach stress reduction that can take the stress out of de-stressing:

CREATE COMMUNITY: Social isolation is a major risk factor for chronic stress, especially for older people, who tend to be more socially isolated. Find a group—a book club, running crew, gardening club, walking group, congregation—any activity that will connect you, ideally in person, to other people. You don't have to become best friends—studies show that just being in the company of other people, even if you don't know them, can have major stress-reducing benefits. If you want the trifecta, exercise with people outside. The combination of exercising in nature with other people has incredible synergy over doing just one (or two) of those things on their own.

BREAK THE CYCLE: Some people deal with stress by drinking too much, binge-eating junk food, staying up late, or getting high—all of which make you more susceptible to viruses. Even though you may think they're helping to relax you, these activities all increase your long-term stress and contribute to a cycle of deteriorating health. If you're struggling with any kind of addiction or harmful behavior, consider seeking out a support group or treatment program for help.

LEAVE IT BEHIND: Learning how to leave a stressful situation behind you after it's over is an important stress management tool. Moving on can be easier said than done, but the relaxation tips and exercises in this section can help you with the transition.

MAKE A SMALL CHANGE: There's no need to make yourself even more stressed out over trying to find the perfect routine to decrease your stress. Find something that works for you, even if it's small, like sitting outside for a few minutes without checking your phone, taking a couple deep breaths, or drinking a cup of tea in silence, and try to do it consistently. The goal is that over time, you'll develop an automatic response when you do that activity that will signal to your brain—and body—that it's time to relax.

LET GO OF TECHNOLOGY: Focus on techniques that don't require a phone, computer, or app, so that you're not dependent on technology and can avoid being distracted. It's fine to explore mindfulness, meditation, deep breathing, yoga, or anything else online, but the goal should be to wean yourself off your device and learn to practice independently.

A PILL IS NOT THE ANSWER: There's no "happy pill" that will make you feel less stressed without some serious side effects. Benzodiazepines like Valium, Xanax, Klonopin, and Ativan, commonly prescribed for anxiety and stress, raise levels of the neurotransmitter GABA (gamma-aminobutyric acid) in your brain, which can have a sedating and calming effect. But in addition to being habit-forming with high risk for abuse, dependence, and a need for escalating doses, these drugs cause cognitive impairment, drowsiness, problems with motor coordination, and amnesia. When you stop taking them, things get even worse: rebound panic and anxiety that can be even more severe than the initial symptoms.

DO WHAT MAKES YOU FEEL GOOD: If there's a particular activity you enjoy doing, such as hiking, walking your dog, reading, listening to music, painting, or anything else that doesn't involve technology and makes you feel happy and relaxed, incorporate that into your regular routine and try to make time for it on a daily basis or as often as you feel you need it. You don't have to do any of the more conventional stress-reducing techniques outlined below. Just go with what feels good in your mind and your body.

As you can see, there are lots of different approaches to reducing stress, but a tried-and-true technique that has been around for a long time involves changing just one critical thing—your response.

The Relaxation Response

The relaxation response is a stress-reducing technique that was popularized in the 1970s at Harvard Medical School by cardiologist

Herbert Benson, although it's been used for centuries by various religious traditions and cultures to alter states of consciousness. The response creates a state of profound rest in your body by slowing your breath, relaxing your muscles, and reducing your blood pressure. It changes your physical and emotional responses to stress and can be elicited in many ways, including meditation, yoga, tai chi, qigong, guided imagery, breath work, prayer, and progressive muscle relaxation. The goal of the relaxation response is to turn down your sympathetic nervous system and activate your parasympathetic nervous system, which causes you to relax. But how exactly do you do that?

Breath focus is one of the most simple ways to elicit the relaxation response, and that's why so many stress-reducing methods are centered around the breath.

Practicing Breath Focus

Breath focus concentrates on slow, deep breathing and helps you disconnect from distracting thoughts and sensations. Here's a simple breathing exercise that you can do on your own without any equipment:

Find a quiet comfortable place to lie down and place one hand on your chest and the other on your abdomen. As you inhale slowly, your bottom hand should move up and out and your top hand and your shoulders should remain relatively quiet. As you exhale, your bottom hand should move back in. (If you're having trouble with this, place a five-pound bag of rice on your abdomen so that you have a physical sensation of where to place the breath.) Now take a slow breath using your chest instead of your abdomen and notice how it produces tension in your neck, shoulders, and back. Now exhale, allowing all of the tension to leave your body. Notice how tension is associated with "chest" breathing and the relaxed feeling you have when you breathe diaphragmatically, that is, when your abdomen moves in and out and your upper body stays quiet.

- Inhale to a slow count of 4 (inflate the abdomen).
- Exhale to a slow count of 6 (deflate the abdomen).
- Modify to a count of 3 for inhalation and 5 for exhalation if that feels more comfortable.

Regardless of the count, your focus should be on exhalation, which should be longer than inhalation by a couple of seconds. Once you've mastered the steps above, you can move on to incorporating a regular practice of controlled breathing into your daily routine. Sit comfortably with your eyes closed. Blend your deep breathing with calming positive imagery and a focus word or phrase that helps you relax. Practice for ten to twenty minutes twice a day, ideally at the same time each day, to establish a ritual and habit, and to truly feel a change in how your body reacts to stress.

Additional benefits of this kind of breath work are that it introduces rich oxygenated air into the lower lobes of your lungs, leads to better lung expansion, and also better brain oxygenation—all very helpful for preventing complications if you do end up becoming infected with a virus.

I've mentioned that honing your stress response shouldn't focus on technology, but here are some apps and devices that can function as training tools to help you develop an effective stress reduction practice:

- Stress thermometer to assess whether your blood vessels are relaxed and dilated
- HeartMath trainer to measure heart rate variability

- Meditation apps like Insight Timer and Headspace
- Breathing apps like Calm and EZ-AIR PLUS

Controlling your stress response isn't just good for your mind; it's an incredibly important part of your anti-viral strategy, since optimizing your stress response optimizes your immune response. You know what else is great for your immune response? A good night's sleep. Being more relaxed and also well rested is a dynamic duo when it comes to achieving the trifecta of improved resistance, enhanced recovery, and better results from vaccination against viruses. Let's find out how to get those z's in.

GET SOME SLEEP!

Even though we know a good night's sleep is critical, many of us miss the mark nightly and still manage to make it through the next day. If you do this often enough, it becomes "normal" for you to feel tired, sluggish, and irritable. You think this is just how you're supposed to feel. In order to really know—not just intellectually, but to feel it in your mind and body—what regular adequate rest can do for you, it's essential to dial in a sleep routine for a few weeks where you're consistently hitting your sleep goals. It's really through the absence of that fatigue, sluggishness, and irritability that you start to understand what you're missing. Good sleep isn't just about feeling (and looking) better—it's a potent anti-viral strategy that will keep your immune system and your entire terrain primed and ready to defend you.

Similar to chronic stress, poor sleep in most people is due to an overactive sympathetic nervous system. Like a computer that won't stop running, your brain stays turned on, even after you try to shut it off, preventing you from switching into sleep mode. There's no shortcut or hack that can replace a good night's sleep—you have to actually put in the hours. But the beauty of sleep is that it's within your grasp, even if you've been a poor sleeper your entire life.

I've divided the recommendations for how to get a restful and restorative night's sleep into five different categories. The more of these guidelines you can adhere to, the better you're likely to start sleeping, but you don't need to do all of them at once. Start with what feels easiest and most accessible and add on from there. You'll know your sleep habits are working when you don't feel sleepy or tired throughout the day and you wake up most days feeling refreshed. Just like exercising and eating a balanced diet, getting a good night's sleep takes practice, but your efforts will pay off with a lifetime of improved health and well-being—plus increased resistance to viruses and infection.

ROUTINE

1) **WIND DOWN:** If you have disordered sleep, there's a high likelihood your sympathetic nervous system's being in overdrive as a result of worry, stress, and anxiety is contributing, so developing a sleep ritual that can help take your mind off whatever's troubling you and get you in the mood for rest is key to restoring sleep. Power-down rituals that you can do about an hour before getting into bed include taking a bath or shower, meditating, drinking herbal tea, reading a book, talking about your day with a member of your household, or listening to calming music. Over time, that routine should signal to your brain—and body—that it's time to shut things down, and the process of falling and staying asleep should become much more automatic.

2) **GET REGULAR:** Your twenty-four-hour circadian rhythm is your internal clock, and it relies heavily on regularity and a

reliable schedule. Going to bed at the same time and waking up at the same time will increase not just the quantity of your sleep but also the quality. It's much better for you to get up at your usual time, even if you feel really tired, than to keep changing your wake-up time to make up for a late night. Remember, regularity trounces length, so resist trying to pay down any sleep debt by oversleeping on the weekends to compensate for not enough during the week. That won't lead to you feeling less tired and more refreshed and will actually make it harder for you to fall asleep at night. Set an ideal sleep schedule and try to stick to it each day.

3) **WRITE IT DOWN:** Write a to-do list and jot down anything else you're concerned about—that can help take concerns and anxieties out of your head and onto the page, allowing your sympathetic nervous system to unload and quiet down. This will help you fall asleep faster, and also fall back asleep if you wake up. Keep the journal by your bed, and if you wake up at night feeling anxious or concerned about something (or with a big idea), get it down in the journal before you try to go back to sleep.

4) **SHUT IT DOWN:** Electronic devices themselves are stimulating, but the content they provide can lead to even more sympathetic activation of your nervous system, moving you in the opposite direction from restful sleep. Limit electronic devices like phones, computers, and tablets for at least an hour before bed. A little television if it's relaxing and not stimulating is okay, but make sure you're not watching it in your bedroom.

5) **AVOID CONFLICT:** Scary movies, disturbing books or podcasts, or getting into arguments just before bedtime can also activate your sympathetic nervous system, create additional stress and worry, and make it more difficult for you to wind down. Try to avoid anything that creates additional stress before bedtime.

6) **AVOID NAPS:** Sleep-pressure chemicals like adenosine build up in your brain during the day, and help you fall asleep at night. Napping can lower adenosine levels and relieve some of that pressure, making it more difficult to fall asleep come bedtime. If you have trouble falling asleep, you should limit daytime naps to under thirty minutes and ideally before lunchtime—or avoid them altogether.

7) **GET SWEATY:** Regular exercise has been scientifically proven to be one of the best ways to relieve stress and anxiety and promote good sleep hygiene. Moderate to vigorous exercise increases sleep quality by reducing the time it takes to fall asleep (sleep onset) and decreasing the amount of time you lie awake in bed at night. Exercise also helps to decrease daytime sleepiness, making it more likely you'll fall asleep easily at night. But keep in mind that strenuous physical activity can also raise endorphin levels, which, in addition to making you feel happy, may also make you feel more alert. To allow your endorphin levels time to fall, try to exercise earlier in the day, or at least two hours before bedtime.

8) **GET ENOUGH:** Take another look at the guidelines on page 87 with the recommended amount of sleep by age. You'll notice that there's a range for each age group. Make your sleep goal the higher number in the range, not the lower one, and keep in mind that you get credit only for the hours you're actually asleep, not from when you get into bed. Although these are recommendations based on scientific study and clinical data, there are always outliers who consistently get less than the recommended amount of sleep, still function well, and are healthy. But if you're one of those people who seems to be perfectly fine on less sleep, you'll never know if you could be even better unless you give getting even more sleep a try.

ENVIRONMENT

9) **MAKE IT COOL:** For sleep to occur, your brain and body have to drop their temperature a few degrees, which is why it's always easier to fall asleep in a cold room than a hot one. Err on the side of having your bedroom feel a little chilly (67°F to 68°F) when you get under the covers. If you don't like feeling cold, wear an extra layer and then strip it off a few minutes after you get into bed or once you start to feel sleepy.

10) **MAKE IT DARK:** The less light your brain senses, the more melatonin (the sleep hormone) it releases. Blackout shades, thick curtains, or even a blanket draped over your windows can help you sleep better at night by decreasing the amount of light being transmitted to your brain through your optic nerve, which will increase melatonin secretion.

11) **LET THE LIGHT IN:** In the morning, let the sun or bright lights into your room so that your brain can sense more light and know it's time to turn off melatonin secretion and wake up and be alert.

12) **VASODILATE:** It may be counterintuitive, but a warm bath or shower actually helps decrease your core body temperature when you get out, due to vasodilation and transfer of heat out of your body through your hands and feet. This can be a great way to help you relax and cool down before bed, but make sure the water is lukewarm and not hot.

13) **MAKE IT HEAVY:** A weighted blanket can help to calm your nervous system and make you feel safer and more secure in bed. But make sure you don't overheat under the weight, which can wake you up and make sleep more difficult.

14) **USE YOUR BEDROOM FOR SLEEP:** Keeping your phone, computer, tablet, or television out of the bedroom helps you avoid using them right before bed, and also helps you to

associate your bed with sleep, and not work, entertainment, or social media.

15) **REMOVE CLUTTER:** Ever notice how calm you feel stepping into a well-appointed hotel room? In addition to comfortable bedding and well-thought-out lighting, most hotel rooms are also uncluttered. There aren't piles of books on the bedside table, heaps of laundry in the corner, or shoes lying around that should be in the closet. For a calming, tranquil sleep environment, keep as few things in your bedroom as possible.

16) **ADD ESSENTIAL OILS:** Lavender, one of the more popular essential oils, is commonly used for relaxation and sleep. Studies have shown that lavender oil can not only help you fall asleep but can also improve the overall quality of rest. Begin diffusing lavender oil an hour or so before turning in for the night.

FOOD/DRINK

17) **EAT SOME TRYPTOPHAN:** Tryptophan, an essential amino acid that cannot be produced by the human body and must be obtained through your diet, primarily from animal- or plant-based protein sources, is a key ingredient in melatonin. Make sure you're getting enough by consuming foods high in tryptophan, which include peanuts, pumpkin and sesame seeds, chicken, eggs, fish, turkey, tofu, and unprocessed non–genetically modified soy.

18) **TRY SOME FERMENTS:** Fermented foods like sauerkraut, kimchi, and even pickled vegetables can improve the health of your microbiome, which helps boost serotonin levels and melatonin production.

19) **AVOID CAFFEINE:** Caffeine has a half-life of several hours, so don't drink any caffeinated beverages past noon—or cut them out altogether. Even though you may think afternoon or

evening caffeine doesn't bother you, studies show it affects everyone's quality of sleep.

20) **LIMIT ALCOHOL:** Alcohol doesn't make you sleepy, it sedates you, and sedation and sleep are not the same thing. Alcohol is a major sleep disrupter, so if you're trying to establish a good sleep routine, reducing or avoiding alcohol is really important. If you are going to drink, limit it to not more than one alcoholic beverage and not within two hours of bedtime. Going to bed tipsy or drunk guarantees poor-quality sleep that night.

21) **DRINK A LITTLE CHERRY JUICE:** Fruit juice, even the unsweetened kind, is on my list of beverages to avoid, but if you're trying to cut down on alcohol, sipping on some tart cherry juice instead can be a helpful substitute. Not only can it simulate the feel and taste of red wine, but tart cherries contain tryptophan and anthocyanins, two compounds that help the body create melatonin and lengthen its effects. Research shows that supplementing with tart cherry juice increases levels of melatonin and helps improve sleep quality and duration. In one study where participants suffering from insomnia drank either 16 ounces of tart cherry juice or the same amount of a placebo juice each day for two weeks, sleep time increased by an average of eighty-five minutes in the cherry juice group. Interestingly, tart cherry juice seems to be just as effective, if not more effective, at reducing insomnia than valerian and melatonin— the two most studied natural products for insomnia.

22) **SIP SOME TEA:** Chamomile and passionflower tea have been found to help with sleep, and the nightly ritual of sipping on a cup of tea can also be soothing. Establish a routine of herbal tea before bedtime, which can become part of your signaling mechanism that it's time to wind down.

23) **EAT EARLY:** Digestion is an active process that can stimulate you and keep you awake. Eating too close to bedtime can also lead to heartburn, which is very disruptive to sleep. Try to finish dinner at least three hours before bedtime and avoid heavy meals at night if you're prone to waking up in the middle of the night.

24) **HYDRATE EARLY:** Try to get most of your liquids in well before bedtime so that you don't wake up multiple times during the night to urinate. Figuring out what your cutoff time is for liquid consumption involves a little bit of trial and error, and depends on bladder capacity, age, and a number of other variables, but pay attention to whether you're getting up at night to pee and move your hydration up accordingly.

MIND-BODY

25) **MEDITATE:** As we discussed in the previous section on stress, a meditation practice is an incredibly effective way to alleviate the worry and anxiety that activate your sympathetic nervous system and lead to stress—and insomnia. Start with just ten slow, deep breaths as part of your wind-down routine and see if you can advance to a longer and deeper pre-bedtime practice.

26) **STRETCH:** Light stretching before bed can help relieve some of the physical and emotional tension that we tend to carry in our bodies. A five- to ten-minute pre-bedtime stretch, accompanied by some slow, easy breathing, can help calm your sympathetic nervous system and get your mind and body relaxed and ready for sleep.

27) **BABY STEPS:** Don't let anxiety and stress about your poor sleep habits disrupt your sleep even more. Small incremental improvements, like getting to bed thirty minutes earlier or

staying off your phone before bed, can have a huge impact, so focus on baby steps that cumulatively will end up making a big difference. And if you get terrible sleep one night, put it behind you and try to do better the next.

28) **BE CAREFUL WITH PILLS:** Small amounts of the sleep supplement melatonin for short periods of time, like with international travel, are probably okay but not advised for long-term use. Studies show that melatonin can help you fall asleep about seven minutes faster and increase your total sleep time by about eight minutes, which are pretty minimal improvements. Because the FDA considers it a dietary supplement, there are no official guidelines for melatonin doses in the United States, but a range of 0.5 milligram to 5 milligrams appears to be safe for most adults, and if you're going to use it, should be taken about one hour before bed. And what about prescription medication? Even though it might be tempting to think that a prescription can help you get a good night's sleep and wake up refreshed in the morning, that's magical thinking. Most sleep aids don't lead to restorative sleep, are habit forming, and leave you groggy and tired the next day, and many of them are associated with cognitive decline if you take them long-term.

. . . . .

Now that you know what to eat and drink, how much exercise you should be getting, ways to shore up your host defenses, stress-reducing techniques, and the recipe for a good night's sleep, let's talk about some environmental factors that you can add to your anti-viral toolbox.

To view the scientific references cited in this chapter, please visit drrobynnechutkan.com/anti-viral-gut-references.

Changing Your Environment

There's a famous eighteenth-century proverb that says, "You must eat a peck of dirt before you die." It refers to the idea that one must endure a certain amount of unpleasantness in life, which is what the dirt represents. But what if it turned out that dirt, rather than being something unpleasant, is actually an essential ingredient for living a healthy life? Let's find out more about how exposure to nature and getting a little dirty can actually help protect you from viruses.

GET OUTSIDE

Fresh air and sunlight don't just make you feel better, they make you better at fighting viruses. A review published in the *Journal of Hospital Infection* in 2019 highlighted an observation made over a century ago and put to use during the Spanish flu epidemic of 1918. The phenomenon is called the open-air factor (OAF) and is defined as the "germicidal constituent in outdoor air that reduces the survival and infectivity of pathogens." In other words: being outside can protect you from infectious organisms. The OAF has been proven to reduce the survival and infectivity of harmful bacteria like *Escherichia coli*, as well as viruses like influenza. In fact, open-air therapy was the standard treatment for infectious diseases like tuberculosis before antibiotics were introduced and is credited with lowering mortality during the Spanish flu epidemic from 40 percent for those recuperating inside, down to 13 percent for those who were put outside in the fresh air to recover.

In addition to handicapping viruses, spending time outside also helps support your immune system. And it's not just fresh air that's helpful. A 2019 study showed that sunlight levels are inversely correlated with influenza transmission. Sunlight is our main source of vitamin D, a vitamin that plays a key role in optimizing our immunity. A 2016 study published in *Nature* found that, separate from its vitamin D–making capabilities, sunlight actually "energizes" T cells, the immune cells that fight infection, and optimizes their response to pathogens.

You might be wondering how you can take advantage of the open-air factor when you're also being encouraged to isolate and stay home. Here are some ideas:

- Spend time outside wherever you have accessible space, including a backyard, front patio, rooftop, or public park.
- Go on hikes, walks, bike rides, and runs in uncrowded areas.
- Do your errands by foot if that's an option.
- Open your windows to bring some fresh air and sunlight in if you're unable to leave home.
- Increase the ventilation in your indoor space to mimic the OAF.

Not only are fresh air and outdoor time important for your immunity, they are also paramount for your mental health in these times of less social interaction. Try to spend at least one hour outside or exposed to fresh air daily, and more if you're able!

Hug a Tree

Spending time outside in the fresh air and also surrounded by trees and nature—a practice the Japanese call "forest bathing," or *shinrin yoku*—is strongly linked to lower blood pressure; a healthier cardiovascular system; decreased anxiety, depression, and fatigue; and enhanced feelings of well-being, happiness, and creativity. Forest bathing has also been clinically shown to accelerate recovery after illness. One mechanism for how spending time in the woods confers benefit is by increasing natural killer cells in our immune system that fight cancer as well as infection. In a study of healthy men published in the *Journal of Biological Regulators and Homeostatic Agents,* both the number and activity of killer cells increased after two-hour walks in a forest park in the Tokyo suburbs, and there was a corresponding drop in stress hormone levels (cortisol and adrenaline) that lasted a full week.

A study of twenty thousand people published in *Nature's Scientific Reports* in 2019 found that spending at least two hours in nature every week was strongly correlated with reporting better health and well-being. Other studies have similarly shown that time spent in nature results in decreased inflammation and enhanced immunity.

Despite knowing that nature is good for you, you may still be having trouble spending enough time in it. (The average person spends almost half the day, a full twelve hours, consuming media or using an electronic device, and the numbers are even higher in teenagers and young millennials.) Forest bathing involves simply walking out into a wooded or forested area (or a park if you're a city dweller), but it can seem a little intimidating if you're not used to doing it. Here are some tips for beginners from the organization Forestry England:

- Turn off your devices to give yourself the best chance of relaxing, being mindful, and enjoying a sensory forest-based experience.
- Slow down. Move through the forest slowly so you can see and feel more.
- Take long breaths deep into the abdomen. Extending the exhalation of air to twice the length of the inhalation sends a message to the body that it can relax.

- Stop, stand, or sit, smell what's around you. What can you smell?
- Take in your surroundings using all of your senses. How does the forest environment make you feel? Be observant. Look at nature's small details.
- Sit quietly using mindful observation; try to avoid thinking about your to-do list or issues related to daily life. You might be surprised by the number of wild forest inhabitants you see using this process.
- Keep your eyes open. The colors of nature are soothing, and studies have shown that people relax best while seeing greens and blues.
- Stay as long as you can. Start with a comfortable time limit and build up to the recommended two hours for a complete forest bathing experience.

Get Dirty

Soil has been essential in the evolution of the human microbiome and provides us with beneficial gut microorganisms, nutrients, genes, and growth-sustaining molecules. Unfortunately, our contact with soil has been greatly reduced, and together with our modern lifestyle and suboptimal diet, this has led to reduced biodiversity in our own internal soil and health effects that include a less able immune system. The good news is that close contact with soil microbes can help to replenish our microbiome, especially when we're also decreasing our consumption of livestock and dairy products and eating a higher diversity of unprocessed organically grown plants.

In addition to spending more time outside in nature, here are some additional dos and don'ts for introducing a little more dirt into your life:

DO visit and purchase your food directly from farms when possible.

DO consider getting a dog, cat, rabbit, or some other pet that will bring a little dirt into your house: children with pets have fewer infections and require fewer antibiotics.

DO let your children get dirty and play on the ground (good for grown-ups, too).

DO consider bathing less often.

DO get your hands dirty by starting a garden. Exposing your immune system to the trillions of microbes in soil is a great way to literally grow a good gut garden.

DO open your windows. Letting nature and aerosolized dirt particles in will improve the health and diversity of the microbes in your home.

DO fill your house with plants for additional soil exposure.

STOP SUPER-SANITIZING

What you do in your daily life has one of two possible effects on your gut shield: strengthening or weakening it. You might not be able to discontinue every potentially damaging habit or practice, but being aware of the risks and making an effort to cut back can still make a difference. With looming viral threats, it can be a fine balance between keeping yourself safe from germs like SARS-CoV-2 and not overutilizing products that strip your body of essential microbes that actually help protect you. Here's some advice on how to navigate that.

Ditch the Hand Sanitizer

Hand sanitizer gels that contain 60 to 80 percent alcohol can be effective in destroying the coronavirus outer layer, but many also possess undesirable ingredients such as triclosan, phthalates, methanol, and parabens that can disrupt your microbiome. If you're in a pinch, I fully support using alcohol-based hand sanitizers (be sure to rub the gel thoroughly into your hands and in between your fingers), but soap and vigorous handwashing with warm water should be your main defensive strategy, because soap is actually more effective than hand sanitizer in completely removing the virus from your skin.

Soaps contain something very special that hand sanitizers don't, and that's "soap molecules." Soap molecules have properties that attract and repel water. When introduced to water, the parts of the molecules that attract water point outward and are able to dissolve lipids (or fats). Lucky for us, the coronavirus is enclosed in a lipid outer layer, which is destroyed during handwashing with soap. Soap also dissolves the weak bonds that hold SARS-CoV-2 together, killing the virus and removing it from your hands. I recommend washing your hands thoroughly with warm water for thirty seconds with an all-natural soap as the gold standard for keeping your hands clean during the pandemic. What about antibacterial soap? Waste of time, since antibacterial soap kills bacteria, not viruses.

Here's a simple and effective healthy soap recipe that you can make at home:

Ingredients
1 cup distilled water
1 cup castile soap liquid
20 drops tea tree essential oil

Method

Add the water to a soap dispenser (you can recycle one that you currently have in your home), then add the castile soap and the tea tree oil. Prior to each use, shake the soap dispenser. Use like regular liquid soap as often as needed.

Here are some additional dos and don'ts that can help you maintain your microbes without going all the way back to the cave:

DO use a chlorine filter for the water you bathe with and drink, since chlorine can damage essential species in your microbiome.

DO stick to mild nonbacterial soaps made from organic non-synthetic oils and use them sparingly just in moist areas like your groin and under your arms, not on the rest of your skin.

DO get a bidet attachment for your toilet so you can rinse your nooks and crannies without having to wash your entire body.

DO use scents made from essential oils instead of alcohol.

DO get sweaty—people who exercise regularly have greater diversity of gut bacteria.

DO make your own natural household cleaner by mixing ½ cup white vinegar with 4 cups of water, 12 drops of tea tree oil, and 12 drops of lavender essential oil. Combine the ingredients in a spray bottle and shake well before using.

DON'T use things *on* your body that you wouldn't put *in* your body. Stick to skin- and hair-care products with simple food-grade ingredients like coconut oil, shea butter, and avocado.

DON'T use soaps, cleansers, or moisturizers that contain petroleum products, FD&C dyes, fragrance, parabens, phthalates, sodium lauryl sulfate, sodium laureth sulfate, triclosan, triethylamine, or other harmful chemicals.

DON'T use shampoos, conditioners, or soaps that contain sodium lauryl sulfate or sodium laureth sulfate, which can make your skin and scalp more sensitive and permeable to toxins.

DON'T use scents containing alcohol that can harm skin microbes.

DON'T use antibacterial soaps and products.

DON'T use mouthwash—it can destroy the microbial ecosystem in your mouth.

Nature is definitely powerful medicine, and getting outside—and a little bit dirty—can do wonders for your microbiome and immune system. But what about actual medicine in your fight against viruses? Are there substances you can take to make you more resilient—and ones you should watch out for? It's all coming up in the next chapter on therapeutics.

To view the scientific references cited in this chapter, please visit
drrobynnechutkan.com/anti-viral-gut-references.

12

Being Thoughtful About Therapeutics

I t's seductive to believe that there's a pill for every ill, but while pharmaceuticals play an important role in many diseases, when it comes to dysbiosis, they're often the cause rather than the cure. With the increasing threat of viral illnesses, now is a good time to take a careful look at some commonly prescribed medications that may be in your medicine cabinet and putting you at risk. It's also a good time to understand the benefits and limitations of probiotics and supplements in improving your gut health. Let's take a deep dive into some of these therapeutics to learn more.

RETHINK THE MEDICINE CABINET

Therapeutics were developed to help what ails us, but while solving one problem, they can often create others. When it comes to preserving the health of your gut microbes, not all drugs are created equal. You need to know which ones are the most problematic and avoid them whenever possible, especially if you already have risk factors for dysbiosis. Antibiotics are clearly at the top of this list, but lots of others, both prescription and over-the-counter medications, can wreak havoc on your microbiome and make you more susceptible to viruses, so the best rule of thumb is to not take a pharmaceutical unless you absolutely have to. In this section I'll go through the top offenders. In addition to telling you what to avoid, I'll provide you with some important questions to ask your health care provider, and suggestions for what to take instead.

Antibiotics

I'm going to focus a lot on antibiotics because they're among the most overprescribed medications, and also the most hazardous to your microbiome. It can be hard to convince people that antibiotics actually make them more prone to infection, since they're designed to treat bacterial infections, but repeated use can actually make pathogens stronger. How does that happen? When exposed to antibiotics, bacteria have a number of ways of surviving attack: they can mutate and become immune; they can produce antibiotic-neutralizing toxins; or they can protect themselves by accessing drug-resistant genes from neighboring bacteria. These resistant "superbug" bacteria like methicillin-resistant *Staphylococcus aureus* (MRSA) kill thousands of people every year in the United States and cause illness in millions more. In fact, antibiotic-resistant infections kill more Americans every year than murders and car accidents combined.

If you take frequent antibiotics when you don't really need them, like for chronic inflammatory conditions like acne or mild infections in your sinuses, urinary tract, or skin that would have resolved on their own without any treatment, you could end up with recurrent (and usually more severe) infections, because of two factors: (1) development of resistant superbugs, and (2) depletion of your essential healthy bacteria that you need to help crowd out pathogens.

Antibiotics have absolutely no activity (zero, zilch, nada) against viruses, including SARS-CoV-2, which causes COVID, and they can actually make you more susceptible to viral illness. The only scenario in which an antibiotic may be helpful for a viral infection is if you're also suffering from a bacterial infection—which can happen due to viral-induced damage to respiratory cells. And who's most at risk for bacterial coinfection? Anyone whose microbial diversity is low and/or has a stable of resistant superbugs as a result of previous antibiotic use.

Remember, a healthy, balanced gut microbiome is your most potent weapon against viruses, so carefully considering the alternatives before you take an antibiotic is a critical part of creating and maintaining an anti-viral gut.

Questions to Ask

If you're suffering from an infection, of course you want to do anything possible to feel better. But taking antibiotics shouldn't be a reflex—it should happen only after thoughtful discussion with your doctor about the pros and cons. Here are five important questions to ask:

1. Is this antibiotic absolutely necessary?
2. Is this antibiotic being prescribed to treat infection or inflammation?
3. If the concern is infection, is it being used to treat an active infection or to prevent one?
4. Are there results from a culture or swab that show this antibiotic will be effective?
5. How likely is this infection to resolve on its own without an antibiotic?

Possible Alternatives

Of course, avoiding an antibiotic altogether is the goal, but if that's not possible, here are some options to ask your health care provider about that will result in less damage to your microbiome:

- A narrow-spectrum antibiotic like penicillin that doesn't kill as many microbes
- A shorter course of antibiotics (three to five days instead of seven to ten days)
- Topical antibiotic formulations like creams, ointments, or drops with fewer systemic effects

So You Have to Take an Antibiotic—Now What?

Your microbiome will take a hit from antibiotics, but it's still possible to mitigate some of the damage by supporting your gut and your microbes during and after. These eight tips will help minimize microbial loss and encourage rapid regrowth:

1. Take a probiotic during and after antibiotics

Even though a probiotic is unlikely to fully reverse the damage of an antibiotic, several studies have documented their usefulness for decreasing side effects like antibiotic-associated diarrhea (AAD) and *Clostridium difficile* (*C. diff*), as well as helping to repopulate the gut. You should start the probiotic at the same time you start the antibiotic, but try to take the probiotic dose at a time as far away from the antibiotics as possible. So, for example, if you're taking an antibiotic twice daily at eight a.m. and eight p.m., you would take the probiotic at two p.m. You should continue the probiotic for at least one month after finishing the course of antibiotics. Probiotics containing various strains of *Lactobacillus* and *Bifidobacteria* are the most useful.

2. Request a narrow-spectrum antibiotic

Taking a narrow-spectrum antibiotic will minimize damage to your microbiome by targeting a narrower range of bacteria. Culture and sensitivity results from urine, stool, sputum, blood, skin, or other body parts (depending on the type and location of infection) will reveal which bacteria are present and which antibiotics they're sensitive to, allowing your doctor to pick a narrow-spectrum antibiotic that will still be effective rather than a broad-spectrum one that will need-lessly kill off additional essential bacteria. Ideally, you should have the culture results before starting treatment so that you know whether your infection is sensitive to the antibiotic you're taking. This can help avoid retreatment with additional courses of antibiotics, as often happens when culture results come back after therapy has already started.

3. Eat prebiotic foods to support your microbiome

Foods high in fiber and resistant starch are important for a healthy microbiome, and they're really critical when you're taking an antibiotic. Not only do they provide food for your microbes, but they also help to promote species diversity, which can decrease dramatically after a course of antibiotics. Fermented foods like sauerkraut and kimchi feed your gut bacteria, and they also provide additional live microbes themselves.

4. Eliminate sugary, starchy foods

Removing these foods from your diet is an essential part of rehabbing your microbiome, and it's particularly important when you're taking an antibiotic. Foods (and drinks) high in sugar and starchy foods that are broken down into simple sugars in the gut send undesirable yeast species into a feeding frenzy, further contributing to microbial imbalance induced by the antibiotics. If you're prone to yeast infections, following a strict anti-yeast diet that excludes any and all sugar while taking antibiotics and for thirty days afterward may be helpful in preventing a flare-up of yeast overgrowth.

5. Eat lots of yeast-fighting foods

Antibiotics are the main cause of yeast overgrowth, which can make you more vulnerable to viruses. But even when you're taking an antibiotic, there are foods you can eat that have significant anti-yeast properties and help combat the yeast-promoting effects of the antibiotics. The list includes onion, garlic, seaweed, rutabaga, pumpkin seeds, and coconut oil. Make sure you're incorporating lots of these foods into your diet while taking antibiotics.

6. Make a mushroom tea

Shiitake and maitake mushrooms have been used as medicine by various cultures throughout the world for thousands of years. They have significant immune-boosting properties and antifungal effects. Chop two dried mushroom caps into small pieces. Add them to a small kettle or pot of water (about 4 cups) and bring to a boil. Reduce the heat, cover, and simmer for about thirty minutes. Strain and serve. You can drink this mushroom tea daily while you're taking antibiotics.

7. Support your liver

Antibiotics, like most drugs, are broken down in the liver, so it's important to make sure that your liver is as healthy as possible while taking them in order to avoid liver damage. Dark green leafy vegetables like kale, spinach, and collard greens, as well as broccoli, beets, and artichokes, can help keep the liver healthy and promote the production of healthy bile. Avoiding alcohol is a must while you are on antibiotics, since it increases the likelihood of liver toxicity.

8. Skip the acid suppression

Blocking stomach acid while you're taking an antibiotic is a recipe for microbial disaster, since the lack of stomach acid leaves you vulnerable to overgrowth of pathogenic bacteria as well as viral attack. If you think you may require an antibiotic, try to stop any acid-suppressing drugs at least seventy-two hours beforehand, and stay off them while you're taking the antibiotic in order to allow levels of stomach acid to return to normal.

Steroids

Unlike antibiotics, which are active against bacteria, steroids work by decreasing inflammation and reducing the activity of your immune system. They're usually reserved for serious inflammatory conditions, like arthritis, autoimmune diseases, or severe allergic reactions. Because of their extensive side effects, including dysbiosis and suppression of your immune system, steroids like prednisone, cortisone, dexamethasone, and others are a major risk factor for viral infections. People taking high dose steroids (more than 20 milligrams per day of prednisone) and/or using them for longer than three months at a time are at the highest risk.

Questions to Ask

The key point with steroids is that the risk is dose dependent and cumulative, so the higher the dose and the longer you take it, the greater the risk. The other thing to know about steroids is that you can't just stop them suddenly; they need to be tapered over a period of time. The main questions to ask are:

1. Is there a lower dose I could take (your goal should be less than 10 milligrams per day of prednisone)?
2. What about taking the steroid every other day instead of daily?
3. Could I try tapering the steroid and then plan to restart it if my symptoms come back?
4. Can you provide me with a tapering schedule?

Possible Alternatives

Consider other non-immunosuppressive anti-inflammatories, less well absorbed formulations, and synthetic forms of steroids that have fewer systemic effects. Here are some options to ask about:

• Anti-inflammatory agents that don't suppress your immune system, like NSAIDs (nonsteroidal anti-inflammatory drugs). Even though NSAIDs are still a problem for your gut, their risk of complications from viral infections is much lower compared to steroids

- Steroid creams or ointments instead of oral steroids
- Synthetic steroids like budesonide that have fewer systemic effects

NSAIDs (Nonsteroidal Anti-inflammatory Drugs)

These medications help relieve fever, pain, and inflammation and include all ibuprofen-containing drugs and aspirin. They're commonly prescribed for muscle and joint pain, as well as headache and other minor ailments, but like many other "wonder drugs," that relief comes at the expense of your gut. NSAIDs increase the intestinal permeability of your gut lining and contribute to the phenomenon of leaky gut, which can potentially allow viruses access to your internal organs.

Questions to Ask

The key things to focus on are keeping the dosage to a minimum, NSAID formulations that are less problematic for the gut, and non-pharmaceutical options for relieving inflammation.

1. A safer dose for the gut is 200 milligrams of ibuprofen or less daily. Would that dose still be effective for my condition?
2. Could I use a different NSAID formulation, like celecoxib (Celebrex) or ketorolac (Toradol), that's less toxic to my gastrointestinal (GI) tract?

Possible Alternatives

- Non-pharmaceutical treatments like ice, massage, physical therapy, acupuncture, etc.
- Acetaminophen (Tylenol) can be problematic for the liver in high doses but is less toxic to the gut than NSAIDs, so it is often a better alternative
- A lower dose of the NSAID plus acetaminophen (Tylenol)

Biologics

These medications have exploded in popularity over the past decade and are prescribed for virtually every autoimmune condition, as well as some forms of inflammation. Although they can be very effective therapeutically, they alter your immune system and lower your ability to fight infections, especially viral ones. If you're on a biologic and are sixty-five years or older, have an already compromised immune system because of a medical condition, or are taking additional immune-suppressing drugs like steroids, you're at especially high risk for viral illness and need to be closely monitored by your doctor for signs and symptoms of infection. Given their risk of infection (and cancer), it's prudent to consider biologics only after other safer drugs as well as diet and lifestyle modifications have been tried.

Questions to Ask

1. Is this drug the only option for treating my condition?
2. Could I lower the dose or lengthen the interval between doses?
3. If my disease is in remission, could I discontinue the medication and restart it if my symptoms flare?

Possible Alternatives

- Anti-inflammatory drugs like 5-aminosalicylates and others that don't have an increased risk of infection
- Biologics to get into remission and then switching to a safer drug as well as dietary and lifestyle modifications to maintain remission

Opioids

These drugs (also known as narcotics) are used to treat a wide range of acute and chronic pain conditions, but as we've seen with the recent opioid epidemic, they're highly addictive, and many people end up using them for much longer than they should. High doses and/or prolonged use over several months can suppress the function of your immune system and may result in end-organ damage that makes you more likely to have a poor outcome from a viral infection. Opioids decrease ventilation in your lungs and increase your risk of viral pneumonia due to effects on your brain's respiratory center. Now is definitely the time to explore nonnarcotic modalities for pain management with your health care provider.

Questions to Ask

1. Is an opioid truly necessary or could I use a nonnarcotic medication for relief of my symptoms?
2. Could a lower dose or a different type of opioid with fewer side effects be substituted?
3. How quickly can I safely taper off this medication?
4. Can you provide me with a tapering schedule and resources to help me discontinue this medication?
5. What should I do if I have withdrawal symptoms?

Possible Alternatives

- Non-pharmaceutical treatments like ice, massage, physical therapy, acupuncture, etc.
- A localized injection of numbing agents, especially for joint or back pain
- Non-opioid prescription drugs like gabapentin and amitriptyline that work on the central nervous system to decrease pain sensation
- Acetaminophen (Tylenol)

Chemotherapy

Chemotherapy refers to various medications that treat cancer. If you have cancer and are on chemotherapy, you should consider taking extra precautions to avoid coming into contact with viruses. In addition to weakening your immune system, certain forms of chemo can cause lung problems like fibrosis and inflammation, which could worsen your prognosis if you get a respiratory viral infection. Discuss timing, length of treatment, number of drugs, and alternatives with your doctor to see if side effects can be minimized, and make sure to eat the most nourishing diet you can while you're on chemo and in the months after, to help your gut recover from the deleterious effects.

Questions to Ask
1. Is it possible to shorten the duration of treatment or decrease the dose of the chemo?
2. I notice my chemo regimen involves multiple drugs. Is it possible to use fewer agents and still get a good result?

Possible Alternatives
If you have cancer, a course of chemotherapy may be unavoidable, but it's still worth asking about alternatives:

- Alternative treatment regimens like photodynamic therapy, laser therapy, immunotherapy, targeted therapy, and hormone therapy that may be effective but not have the same immune-suppressing effects
- Natural remedies to decrease the toxicity of the chemotherapy on your immune system and microbiome

Hormones
Birth control pills (BCPs) are one of the most common forms of contraception and are also prescribed to decrease menstrual cramps, clear up acne, treat endometriosis, and reduce symptoms of premenstrual syndrome. Unfortunately, both BCPs and hormone replacement

therapy (HRT) used to treat menopausal symptoms affect your microbial ecosystem and can lead to dysbiosis. But messing with your microbiome isn't the only problem with these drugs; they're also associated with an increased risk for blood clots, which can be an important complication of viral illnesses like COVID—causing rashes, breathing problems, heart attacks, and strokes. The likelihood of your BCP or HRT causing blood clots is pretty low, but if you're taking one of these drugs and are over fifty, obese, a smoker, or have a history of underlying clotting disorders, heart disease, high blood pressure, or previous blood clots or stroke, you may be at increased risk and should talk to your health care provider about whether it's safe to continue taking them.

Questions to Ask
1. Do you think it's safe for me to continue taking this medication given the current viral threat and the possibility of clotting complications?
2. Would it be appropriate to lower the dose of the medication to decrease my risk of blood clots?
3. Is there a medication that has a lower risk of blood clots that would be advisable for me to take instead?

Possible Alternatives
- Nonhormonal methods of birth control like condoms, a nonhormonal copper intrauterine device (IUD), a cervical cap, or a diaphragm
- Topical HRT applied to the skin in the form of patches and gels that don't carry a risk of blood clots
- Natural therapies for menopausal symptoms like black cohosh, unprocessed soy, flaxseed, vitamin E, yoga, breathing exercises, a plant-based diet, cold drinks, cutting back on alcohol

Proton Pump Inhibitors (PPIs)
See Chapter 9 ("Securing Defenses").

CONSIDER A PROBIOTIC

Before we dive into the details of which type of probiotic may be helpful in combating viruses, let's start with a few definitions:

> **Probiotics** are live microorganisms that provide a health benefit to the host, usually ingested in pill, powder, or liquid form. When we talk about probiotics, we are generally referring to microorganisms in a supplement, not the native microbes in your gut.
> **Prebiotics** are foods or ingredients that promote the growth of beneficial bacteria in the digestive tract. In other words, they're food for your gut bacteria.
> **Postbiotics** are compounds made when bacteria in your gut digest and break down prebiotic fibers.

Just as antibiotics don't have any direct activity against viruses, probiotics don't, either. That being said, they can be helpful for safeguarding against viral infections via several mechanisms, including improving the diversity and composition of your microbiome, maintaining the integrity of your intestinal barrier, producing active metabolites that have anti-viral capabilities, and most important, enhancing your immune response.

Despite their potential usefulness, one of the challenges with evaluating probiotics is that they fall under the category of supplements, so they aren't regulated by the Food and Drug Administration in the United States. This means that a probiotic pill may not actually contain the amounts of bacteria listed on the label, or the bacteria may not be alive and active. People often institute other healthy diet and lifestyle changes when starting a probiotic or are biased to believe that the probiotic will be helpful, making it even more challenging to figure out whether it's truly making a difference.

While there aren't a ton of randomized placebo controlled trials (the gold standard for scientific investigation) that have studied the benefits of probiotics for combating viruses, we have clinical data for probiotics containing strains of *Lactobacillus* and *Bifidobacteria* that show usefulness in combating rotavirus, influenza, and viral gastroenteritis. In clinical trials, administering certain combinations of high-dose probiotics to hospitalized COVID patients resulted in lower rates of needing a ventilator, ICU admission, and death. It's important to note that these are probiotic cocktails that aren't available off the shelf to the general public and are administered in a monitored setting by medical professionals.

Common Probiotic Strains

Here are some common strains of bacteria that are generally helpful for remediating dysbiosis and found in many popular brands of probiotics:

> *Lactobacillus acidophilus* ferments sugars into lactic acid and produces amylase, which helps digest carbohydrates. It's one of the most popular probiotics and is used commercially in many dairy products. It's highly resistant to stomach acid and adheres well to intestinal cells, helping to prevent the proliferation of opportunistic species—essentially taking up all the barstools so bad bacteria can't get a drink.
>
> *Lactobacillus casei* is found in the mouth and intestines, and also in fermented vegetables, milk, and meat. It has shown efficacy in combination with other strains in alleviating GI

conditions such as antibiotic-associated and infectious diarrhea, as well as in respiratory tract infections.

Lactobacillus rhamnosus is very hardy and resistant to stomach acid and bile. It's present in the mouth and in the GI tract, and also in the vagina and urinary tract of women, where it can prevent pathogens from gaining a foothold. *L. rhamnosus* has been used successfully to treat diarrhea caused by rotavirus, as well as influenza and viral pneumonia. Despite its many uses as a probiotic, it's been associated with infection in people with a weakened immune system.

Lactobacillus salivarius suppresses pathogenic bacteria and reduces gas in people with irritable bowel syndrome (IBS).

Bifidobacterium bifidum is part of the normal flora of the large intestine and also one of the most common probiotics. It helps break down and absorb simple sugars and has been shown to aid immune function by decreasing the severity of symptoms and the length of illness from viruses that cause the common cold.

Bifidobacterium longum is one of the founding species in infants, and it thrives in the low-oxygen environment of the colon. It helps prevent the growth of pathogens by producing lactic acid, and can also improve lactose tolerance, prevent diarrhea, and ameliorate allergies.

Bifidobacterium lactis is also known as *B. animalis*. Its beneficial effects on abdominal discomfort and bloating in people with constipation-predominant IBS are well described, and in clinical trials it was shown to protect intestinal cells from damage by gluten in people with celiac disease.

How to Choose a Probiotic

Although there's no one-size-fits-all version when it comes to probiotics, here's some general advice for choosing a probiotic:

- Probiotics on the market generally contain from one billion to nine hundred billion colony forming units (CFUs). Pick one with at least fifty billion CFUs of the two most important groups of probiotic bacteria: *Lactobacilli* and *Bifidobacteria.*
- Most robust probiotics contain several different bacterial strains designed to work together, since different strains have different functions and no one strain can provide all the benefits.
- Choose a probiotic with enteric coating to protect the bacteria from being destroyed by stomach acid.
- Make sure the product has a good safety record with regard to human use. Check trusted sites on the internet to see whether any clinical trials or other scientific studies have been done to assess side effects, or whether the manufacturer provides any safety information.
- Check to see what the shelf life is, whether the product needs to be refrigerated (most of the better ones do), and whether it's stable under normal storage conditions.
- The manufacturer should guarantee that the product was tested and certify that it contains the amount of live bacteria stated on the label. This should be on the package label or insert.

The probiotic I use the most in my practice is Visbiome, which contains eight strains of live bacteria and is considered a high-potency medical food. The definition of a medical food is: "a food which is formulated to be consumed or administered under the supervision of a physician and which is intended for the specific dietary management of a disease or condition for which distinctive nutritional require-ments, based on recognized scientific principles, are established by medical evaluation." Unlike regular supplements, medical foods are regulated by the U.S. Food and Drug Administration.

Visbiome is scientifically formulated to promote gut health and is backed by over twenty years of research and almost a hundred scientific studies. In addition to the vast amount of research behind the product, I use it because I find it clinically helpful in my patients with inflammatory bowel disease, IBS, dysbiosis, and other gut-based conditions. Of course, like any probiotic, it's most effective when used in conjunction with dietary change.

Limitations and Risks of Probiotics

Probiotics have a pretty good safety record, but, as with any therapeutic, there can be risk involved. Formulations can become contaminated with harmful strains, and in someone who has a compromised immune system, even benign bacteria in the formulation can be a hazard. Transfer of harmful genes and overstimulation of the immune system are rare but are among the more serious potential side effects. For the average person, side effects are usually mild and include gas, bloating, nausea, and occasionally diarrhea. When I prescribe a probiotic, I'll usually tell my patients to start with a quarter or half dose and increase gradually to the full amount over three to four weeks so that their body has time to get used to it.

Even if a probiotic has the amount of bacteria it claims to have, there's no guarantee that these bacteria will actively colonize your gut and result in a change in your microbiome, so while it may still make sense to take one, don't forget to ramp up your fiber intake to feed your existing gut bacteria, and avoid microbe-depleting drugs like antibiotics whenever possible.

BE REALISTIC ABOUT SUPPLEMENTS

Almost every supplement these days claims to be good for your microbiome or states that it can boost your immune system in some way, but relying on natural forms of these ingredients from food is always best, and that's where we have the most data to support beneficial effects. For example, you can get tons of vitamin C from citrus, bell peppers, strawberries, and tomatoes; vitamin D from fish and eggs (and sunlight); and vitamin E from almonds, spinach, broccoli, and olive oil.

The other thing to keep in mind when it comes to supplementation is that association does not necessarily mean causation. Vitamin D deficiency has been associated with a number of different viral diseases including influenza, HIV, hepatitis C, and COVID, but that doesn't mean that supplementing with vitamin D will make you less susceptible to those viruses. People who are in poor health often have micronutrient deficiencies, so it's not surprising that low vitamin levels are associated with a wide range of diseases, including cancer, autoimmune diseases, and viral infections.

Bottom line: there is no miracle cure-all supplement that can make you healthy. You have to put in the work with your diet and lifestyle if you're trying to reap the benefits. But while getting the nutrients you need from food is the goal, not everyone has access to these healthy foods all the time or is able to eat them in sufficient quantities, and supplementing can sometimes help bridge any deficits.

Keeping yourself safe from viruses involves addressing dysbiosis, so let me tell you about a few supplements that may be helpful for your microbiome—especially when used in conjunction with a diet rich in plant fiber. Some work by inhibiting unhealthy bacteria, while others boost levels of beneficial species or have antiparasitic, antifungal, or anti-viral effects. Here are some you should know about:

SUPPLEMENTS THAT MAY BE USEFUL IN TREATING DYSBIOSIS

Berberine—active against *Candida albicans* and *Staphylococcus aureus*

Enteric-coated peppermint oil—helpful in small intestinal bacterial overgrowth (SIBO) and IBS

Garlic—active against bacteria, fungi, viruses, and parasites

Glutamine—may be helpful for repairing the lining of the gut in dysbiosis and leaky gut

Grapefruit seed extract—has antimicrobial and antifungal activity

Inulin—fermentable fiber with prebiotic properties that increases growth of beneficial bacteria

Olive leaf extract—has anti-inflammatory and antibacterial effects

Oregano oil—good for nail fungus and sinus infections; also has antiparasitic effects

Psyllium husk—plant-based fiber with prebiotic and stool-bulking properties

Tea tree oil—has natural antifungal properties

Turmeric/curcumin—has anti-inflammatory properties and improves immune function

Zinc—may enhance barrier function of the gut

There's no magic wand for quickly and reliably undoing damage to your gut microbiome or optimizing your immune system, although, over time, removing harmful medications, replacing depleted species, and making sure your micronutrient requirements are covered can help. Probiotics and supplements aren't a panacea, but in conjunction with meaningful dietary change, they may provide some added benefit to your anti-viral capabilities.

. . . . .

Now that you know what you should be doing to strengthen your gut shield, let's take a peek at what a day in the life of an anti-viral gut looks like.

To view the scientific references cited in this chapter, please visit

drrobynnechutkan.com/anti-viral-gut-references.

13

Plan at a Glance

I don't worry much about becoming infected with a virus. That
doesn't mean I won't get sick, but I channel any negative energy and
anxiety about my health into positive actions that move me toward
my goal of not getting sick. My system (my daily habits) support my
goal (not getting sick). As James Clear explains in his bestselling book
Atomic Habits, your system is what you do every day to get to your
goal. Put another way, "fix the inputs and the outputs will take care of
themselves." When it comes to my goal of not getting sick from a
virus, my system is a pretty simple "dirt, sweat, veg" routine: I try to
get outside in nature every day, work up a good sweat, and make sure
I'm eating lots of vegetables. I don't worry about the details—like how
long I'm outside for, or whether I'm in the woods or just walking
around the neighborhood, or what kind of exercise I'm doing, or how
the vegetables are prepared. My system is just to make sure that I'm
hitting all three on a daily basis. Of course, there are other things I do,
too, like paying attention to how much sleep I'm getting and my alcohol consumption, but *dirt, sweat, veg* are my ride or die guidelines.

One of the things I've noticed during this pandemic is that many
people are looking for a "hack" to protect them from viral infection.
We can all improve our resilience to viruses, and while I've given you
a wide range of interventions that can help you do that, it's not any
one of those things on its own that truly moves the needle; it's

figuring out a system to help you incorporate the most essential ones consistently on a daily basis. Those small things you do every day add up to big changes in your ability to protect yourself from viral illness—but you have to actually do them.

While the preceding chapters provided more specific details, let me give you a snapshot of what a day in the life of an anti-viral gut looks like by sharing my top 10 list of things to do (or not do) every day to move you toward your goal of resisting viruses.

MY TOP 10 LIST

EAT MORE VEGETABLES

Doesn't matter if they're raw, steamed, sautéed, or blended up in a smoothie—just get them in, because they're essential food for your army of gut bacteria. If you're having trouble, use my 1-2-3 rule to get to at least six servings a day. And remember that variety is important for providing your microbes with an array of nutrients, so keep that goal of thirty different plant foods a week in mind.

PASS ON FACTORY FOOD

If it's in a box, bag, packet, or pouch with a label and a list of ingredients (especially ones you can't pronounce that sound like a science experiment), put it down and pick up something that came off a tree, off a bush, or out of the ground instead. Preferably with a little dirt on it!

INCLUDE SOME FERMENTS

Just one tablespoon of sauerkraut contains up to one billion live bacteria, over two dozen distinct strains that can help repopulate your gut, plus the fiber to feed them. Have a small (or large!) serving of these medicinal foods every day.

DRINK ALCOHOL IN MODERATION—OR NOT AT ALL

Make sure you're not exceeding 0 to 14 drinks per week if you're a man, and 0 to 7 if you're a woman. Keep in mind that "none" may be easier to navigate than "some," so if you're struggling to moderate your drinking, consider whether it may actually be easier to give it up altogether.

HYDRATE

Drink at least half your body weight in ounces of plain old water every day, in addition to any other beverages. Keep an eye on your pee and make sure it's not too yellow, which can be a sign that you need to up your water intake even more.

AVOID UNECESSARY MEDICATIONS

Don't take medications that aren't absolutely necessary, since so many drugs mess up your microbiome or damage your gut lining (or both!). Be especially cautious with antibiotics, acid blockers, immunosuppressive drugs like steroids, and NSAIDs (nonsteroidal anti-inflammatory drugs). Review your medication regularly with your health care provider and ask about alternatives, a lower dose, or discontinuing it altogether.

SLEEP

Establish a regular sleep routine of seven to nine hours of uninterrupted sleep nightly and try to get into and out of bed at around the same time every day, even on the weekends.

EXERCISE

Work up a sweat by moving your body for at least half an hour five days/week or more. Even if you're not actually sweating, try to exercise vigorously enough to make it difficult to speak comfortably in full sentences.

GET OUTSIDE

Spend some time outside in nature every day, even if it just means sitting on a patch of grass or walking around the block. Try to keep this up even if the weather isn't great or you really don't feel like it.

GET QUIET

Find a little time every day to do absolutely nothing except for some deep breathing or quiet meditation. How, where, when, and how long you do this for will depend on your schedule, environment, and personal preference, but set an intention to doing this regularly and build from there.

. . . . .

You can't control what's going on in the world, but you can control what's going on in the inner world of your terrain. Manage the small, simple, essential things that add up to make a big difference. Work on your inputs so you can reap the output of increased resilience to viruses.

To view the scientific references cited in this chapter, please visit
drrobynnechutkan.com/anti-viral-gut-references.

14

Recipes
All recipes by Elise Museles

My goal with these recipes is to help you assemble simple, delicious, microbe-boosting food with minimum effort and maximum taste. These are dishes you can eat anytime, for any meal. Mix and match as you see fit (sort of like a capsule wardrobe approach) and serve them up on their own or as a side dish to accompany whatever else is on the table. One thing you'll notice is that while these recipes aren't all strictly vegan, they're overwhelmingly plant-based with tons of fiber to feed your microbes, and none of them contain processed carbohydrates, refined sugar, dairy, gluten, or large amounts of animal protein. Don't feel like following the recipes exactly? No problem! Use the ingredient lists as a guide to inspire you to get more plants in. And if one of my dishes ends up on your plate next to something that's not quite as good for your gut, that's okay, too; just make that portion a little smaller and mine a little bigger and it will all work out.

FOOD CATEGORIES
Soups
Everything but the Kitchen Sink Soup

Lentil Soup

Quick Chicken Soup with Brown Rice

White Beans and Greens Soup

Immunity Vegetable Broth

Smoothies

Dr. Chutkan's Gutbliss
   Green Smoothie
Blueberry Bliss Smoothie
Tropical Green Smoothie
Healing Orange-Ginger Smoothie
Chocolate Raspberry Dessert
   Smoothie

Salads

GUIDE: How to Build a Salad
   That Keeps You Satisfied and
   Feeling Good
Cabbage-Kale Crunch
Root Vegetable Salad with Herby
   Vinaigrette
Arugula Salad with Quinoa,
   Avocado, Blueberries, and
   Walnuts
Grilled Peach and White Bean Salad
   with Basil Vinaigrette
Beet, Fennel, and Orange Salad
   with Cumin Lime Dressing

Hearty One-Pot Dishes

Moroccan Spiced Chickpeas
Cauliflower Tikka Masala
Mexican Spiced Quinoa
   Vegetable Stew
Lentils and Roasted Carrots with a
   Lemon-Herb Tahini Sauce
Skillet Shakshuka

Ferments

Fermented Veggie Guide
Easy Coconut Milk Kefir

Snacks

Lemony Garlic Hummus
High-Fiber Trail Mix
Root Veggie Chips with Tahini
   Dipping Sauce
Two-Way Sweet Potato Toasts

Desserts

Zesty Chia Pudding
"Cookie Dough" Balls
Chocolate Orange Mousse
Skillet Peach Crisp

SOUPS

———

Everything but the Kitchen Sink Soup
Serves 8

With more than fifteen different veggies and herbs, this soup will get you more than halfway to your goal of thirty different plant foods per week—in just one bowl of soup!

Ingredients

2 tablespoons olive oil or avocado oil

1 yellow or sweet onion, diced

1 garlic clove, minced

3 celery stalks, diced

4 carrots, diced

1 teaspoon dried oregano

1 teaspoon dried parsley

4 cups vegetable broth, plus more as needed

1½ cups cooked cannellini or great northern beans or 1 (15-ounce) BPA-free can, drained and rinsed

1 (28-ounce) can diced tomatoes (or equivalent fresh tomatoes, chopped)

1 (6-ounce) can tomato paste

6 cups vegetables, chopped (broccoli, red pepper, yellow squash, zucchini, green beans, cauliflower, etc.)

3 cups fresh spinach leaves (reserve until the end)

2 tablespoons fresh parsley

Sea salt and freshly ground black pepper to taste

Crushed red pepper flakes (optional for an additional kick)

Method

Heat the oil in a large pot over medium-high heat. Add the onion, garlic, celery, and carrots. Sauté until lightly browned. Add in the oregano and parsley to coat the vegetables. Next, add the vegetable broth, beans, tomatoes, and tomato paste. Mix thoroughly and then place the chopped vegetables in the pot. Add enough water or additional broth to cover the vegetables. Bring to a boil over high heat, then reduce the heat to a simmer, cover, and cook for 35 to 40 minutes, until the vegetables are soft.

Remove from the heat and add the spinach leaves. Place the lid back on the pot for 5 minutes to allow the spinach to steam. Season with salt and pepper. Add red pepper flakes if desired.

———

Lentil Soup
Serves 6

This super simple soup loaded with MACs (microbiota-accessible carbohydrates) is manna for your microbes.

Ingredients
2 tablespoons olive oil

1 medium yellow onion, chopped

2 large stalks celery, chopped

2 large carrots, chopped

2 or 3 garlic cloves, minced

1 teaspoon ground turmeric

½ teaspoon ground cumin

1½ teaspoons dried oregano

1 cup chopped tomatoes (from a can or carton if fresh not available)

4 cups low-sodium vegetable broth

1 cup brown or green lentils, rinsed

1 teaspoon sea salt, plus more as needed

Freshly ground black pepper, plus more as needed

2 tablespoons fresh parsley, chopped

3 cups fresh spinach or other leafy greens

1½ tablespoons freshly squeezed lemon juice (or juice from
    ½ large lemon)

Crushed red pepper flakes (optional)

Method

In a large pot over medium-high heat, heat the olive oil. Add the onion and sauté for 5 to 6 minutes, until almost translucent. Add the celery, carrots, garlic, turmeric, cumin, and oregano to the pot and stir continuously for 8 minutes. Add the tomatoes with their juice and cook for a few more minutes.

Add the broth, lentils, salt, and black pepper. Bring the soup to a boil over high heat. Reduce the heat to medium-low. Cover and simmer for 45 to 60 minutes, until the lentils are softened. Stir in the parsley, the greens, and the lemon juice. Season the soup with additional salt, black pepper, and crushed red pepper flakes, if using. Ladle into bowls for a plant-powered meal.

Quick Chicken Soup with Brown Rice
Serves 6

In addition to chicken, this hearty soup has lots of veggies and seasonings. Use quinoa instead of brown rice or play around with a variety of fresh herbs.

Ingredients

1½ tablespoons avocado oil or olive oil

½ cup chopped onion

2 garlic cloves

1 tablespoon fresh ginger, grated, or 1 teaspoon ground

1 tablespoon fresh turmeric, grated, or 1 teaspoon ground

3 large carrots, sliced into rounds

2 stalks celery, chopped

1 parsnip, peeled and sliced into rounds

6 cups chicken or vegetable broth

1 pound skinless, boneless chicken breasts

1 sprig of fresh thyme

1 sprig of fresh rosemary, plus extra for garnish

1 teaspoon sea salt, or to taste

Freshly ground black pepper to taste

½ cup uncooked brown rice

Method

Heat the oil in a large pot over medium-high heat. Add the onion, garlic, ginger, and turmeric and sauté for 3 to 5 minutes, until soft. Then add the carrots, celery, and parsnips and sauté for an additional 3 to 4 minutes, until soft. Add the broth, chicken breasts, thyme, rosemary, salt, and pepper.

Bring the soup to a boil over high heat and pour in the brown rice. Once boiling, stir to cover the mixture with liquid, then reduce the heat to low. Cover and simmer for 40 to 45 minutes, until the chicken is cooked through and the rice is soft.

Remove the chicken from the pot and place it on a cutting board. Shred it into bite-sized pieces and return the shredded chicken to the pot. Stir. Adjust the seasonings and add more broth if desired for a thinner consistency. Garnish with fresh rosemary and serve immediately.

———

White Beans and Greens Soup

Serves 4

With a bright, bold flavor and a big dose of plant-based protein and fiber, a bowl of this soup is a memorable meal on its own.

Ingredients

1½ pounds fresh tomatillos (see Note)

2 poblano or Anaheim peppers

1 medium to large jalapeño pepper

1 teaspoon olive oil

Fine sea salt

4 whole garlic cloves, peeled

1 medium yellow onion, sliced

4 cups low-sodium vegetable broth, plus more as needed

½ cup chopped fresh cilantro, plus extra for garnish

1½ teaspoons ground cumin

1½ teaspoons dried oregano

Freshly ground black pepper

2 (15-ounce) cans cannellini beans, drained and rinsed, or 3 cups
     cooked beans

2 cups fresh baby spinach

1 large ripe avocado, peeled, pitted, and sliced

1 lime, cut into wedges

Sliced radish and red pepper flakes, for garnish (optional)

Method

Position an oven rack 6 to 8 inches below the broiler and preheat the broiler. Line a rimmed baking sheet with parchment paper.

Husk the tomatillos. Rinse the tomatillos, poblano, and jalapeño, then pat them dry. Place them on the prepared baking sheet. Drizzle with the olive oil. Sprinkle with salt and toss to coat evenly. Drizzle the garlic cloves with a little oil and wrap them in a small piece of parchment before placing them on the baking sheet.

Broil for about 10 minutes, until the tomatillos and peppers start to char. Add the onions to the baking sheet and drizzle with a little oil. Turn the peppers and broil for 5 to 10 minutes longer, until charred and tender. Set aside to cool.

Discard the stems and seeds from the peppers (leave the seeds in the jalapeño if you want a spicier soup) and unwrap the garlic cloves. Place the roasted tomatillos, peppers, onion, garlic, 1 cup of the broth, cilantro, cumin, and oregano in the bowl of a food processor or blender and puree until mostly smooth, or use an immersion blender in a saucepan.

Pour the mixture into a medium saucepan and add the remaining 3 cups of broth. Taste and adjust the seasoning with salt and black pepper. Add the beans. Bring to a boil over high heat, then reduce the heat to low and simmer, partially covered, for about 20 minutes, until the mixture cooks down a little. Add the spinach and stir until the spinach is wilted. If you like a thinner soup, add a little more broth. Ladle into bowls and top with avocado and cilantro. Serve with lime wedges on the side, as well as the radishes and crushed red pepper flakes, if using.

Note

Can't find fresh tomatillos? Use an 11-ounce can of whole tomatillos, but don't roast them—just drain and add to the bowl of the food processor with the other roasted vegetables.

Tips
Add another jalapeño for a spicier soup.

Substitute chopped kale, chard, or other greens for the spinach; adjust the cooking times as needed to make sure the greens are tender.

————

Immunity Vegetable Broth
Makes 3 quarts

Add in additional vegetables like leeks, shallots, fennel bulbs, and parsnips—all of which blend in nicely with the flavor of this nourishing soup and provide more nutrients for you and your microbes.

Ingredients
3 stalks celery, coarsely chopped
2 large carrots, coarsely chopped
1 yellow onion, coarsely chopped
6 ounces cremini mushrooms, coarsely chopped
3 ⅛-inch-thick slices fresh ginger
2 teaspoons peeled and grated fresh turmeric
2 garlic cloves, smashed
½ teaspoon fine sea salt
½ teaspoon coarsely ground black pepper

Method
Add all of the ingredients to an Instant Pot (ideally 6-quart size). Add 2 quarts water and stir to combine. Secure the lid and set the Pressure Release to Sealing. Select the Soup/Broth setting and set the cooking time for 30 minutes at high pressure.

Once the Instant Pot cooking cycle is complete, let the pressure release naturally for at least 20 minutes, then move the Pressure Release to Venting to release any remaining steam.

Alternatively, add all of the ingredients plus 2 quarts water to a large stockpot, bring to a boil over high heat, then reduce the heat to low, cover, and simmer for 1 hour.

Place a fine-mesh strainer over a large bowl and strain the broth into the bowl. Discard the solids or skip this step for a big fiber boost. Let cool completely. Store in airtight containers in the refrigerator for up to 1 week or in the freezer for future use.

SMOOTHIES

Dr. Chutkan's Gutbliss Green Smoothie
Serves 2 to 3

This nutrient-dense smoothie will help you get to that magical number of six to eight servings of green vegetables per day that corresponds to meaningful changes in your microbiome. Probiotics can help to add beneficial bacterial species to your gut, but in order to achieve colonization and repopulation you need to consume large amounts of indigestible plant fiber to feed those microbes. A green smoothie every day is a great way to accomplish this. Be sure to use fresh, locally grown, organic produce, include the fibrous stalks/stems of the vegetables, and add plenty of liquid so it's not too thick (it should be the consistency of pulpy orange juice).

You can make this smoothie just using one of the recommended base liquids and some greens, but for a more palatable taste add some herbs and/or spices and fruit.

Ingredients

Base

Water, or unsweetened and unflavored coconut water, or brewed
    unsweetened herbal tea
Ice for desired consistency

Greens

1 handful each (about 1 packed cup) of kale, collards, spinach, chard, or
   any other leafy green (pick two or three)
1 stalk celery

Herbs/Spices

Small bunch of fresh parsley or mint or cilantro (optional)
½-inch piece of fresh ginger (optional but helpful for gut motility)

Fruit

Small green apple, pear, peach, or nectarine, or 1 kiwi, or ½ cup pineapple
   or mango, or ½ cup berries (optional—pick one or two)
Juice of ½ lemon (optional)

Method

Place all of the ingredients in a Vitamix or other high-speed blender and
blend well. Drink immediately after blending. You can refrigerate any
extra for consumption within 24 hours, but you'll need to reblend or stir the
smoothie vigorously because the ingredients will start to separate. Cheers!

Blueberry Bliss Smoothie

Serves 1 to 2

Try blackberries, raspberries, or strawberries in place of the blueberries
or use a combination of all four. Play around with different leafy greens
to get a variety of nutrients and flavors. Think kale or romaine lettuce, to
name a few!

Ingredients

1 cup plant-based milk, plus more as needed
2 heaping handfuls of fresh spinach or leafy greens of choice
¼ large avocado
1 cup frozen blueberries
½ to 1 frozen banana
Pinch of sea salt

Method

Add the milk, spinach, and avocado to the bowl of a blender and blend until well combined. Mix in the blueberries, banana, and salt. Blend until smooth and creamy, adjusting the liquid if necessary.

———

Tropical Green Smoothie
Serves 1 to 2

Toss in 1 or 2 tablespoons of hempseeds to add an extra dose of protein and healthy fats.

Ingredients

1 cup coconut water (use coconut milk for a creamier smoothie), plus more
    as needed
2 tablespoons fresh cilantro
1 handful of fresh spinach
¼ large avocado
1½ cups fresh or frozen pineapple
1 teaspoon lime zest
1 teaspoon lime juice
Pinch of sea salt

Method

Add the coconut water, cilantro, spinach, and avocado to the bowl of a blender and blend until well combined. Mix in the pineapple, lime zest, lime juice, and salt and blend until smooth and creamy, adjusting the liquid if necessary.

———

Healing Orange-Ginger Smoothie
Serves 1 to 2

Not a mango fan? Try sliced and frozen pear instead. You can also use regular steamed, then frozen cauliflower in place of the cauliflower rice. Just make sure to add some kind of vegetable for the fiber and anti-viral nutrients.

Ingredients

1 cup coconut water (use coconut milk for a creamier smoothie), plus more
    as needed

1 orange, peeled, segmented, and frozen

½ cup mango, cubed and frozen

¼ cup cauliflower rice, frozen

½ teaspoon ground turmeric

½-inch slice of fresh ginger, peeled

Method

Add the coconut water, orange, mango, cauliflower rice, turmeric, and
ginger to the bowl of a blender. Blend until well combined, adjusting the
liquid if necessary.

———

Chocolate Raspberry Dessert Smoothie
Serves 2

You can use any type of berries in this decadent blend or take it in a
different direction and use frozen orange slices in place of the raspberries.
It will taste completely different without compromising any of the
nutritional benefits.

Ingredients

1 cup plant-based milk, plus more as needed

1 banana, sliced and frozen

1 cup raspberries, frozen

1 handful of fresh spinach

2 tablespoons raw cacao or cocoa powder

½ teaspoon vanilla extract

Pinch of sea salt

Method

Add the milk, banana, raspberries, spinach, cacao, vanilla, and salt to the
bowl of a blender. Blend until smooth and creamy, adjusting the liquid if
necessary.

SALADS

GUIDE: How to Build a Salad That Keeps You Satisfied and Feeling Good

Contrary to popular belief, salads can be filling and satisfying. They provide you with lots of fiber and important nutrients, and connect you to food straight from the earth. Committing to a salad every day is a great way to incorporate more plants into your meals, especially fresh vegetables, fruit, nuts, legumes, seeds, and herbs. Here are some foolproof methods to up your salad game and move beyond boring bowls of wilted lettuce:

- Instead of getting stuck on a list of ingredients, **stick to the season**. Mother Nature knows what's best when it comes to giving our bodies what they need at just the right time. Think hydrating and lighter foods like tomatoes, cucumbers, and melons in the spring and summer, and heartier foods such as root veggies in the fall and winter.

- **Prep planning** is key for quick and easy assembly, and it doesn't have to be complicated. Chop your raw veggies and roast or grill a batch, too. Or just leave your ingredients washed and ready to eat. Then store them in the fridge to mix and match all week.

- **Include a balance** of protein (this can be animal or vegetable) and healthy fats (think nuts, seeds, avocado) for sustained energy, balanced blood sugar, and to fill you up.

- **Texture and crunch** are essential for satisfaction. Roasted chickpeas, almonds, walnuts, sunflower seeds, carrots, celery, and snap peas all do the trick—and are ideal foods to feed your microbes.

- A little fruit in your salad can **help satisfy a sweet tooth**. Try fresh berries, peaches, or pineapple for a fun, fruity kick.

- If you run out of ideas, **pick themes** that go together for inspiration: Asian, Mexican, Greek, Thai, Moroccan to name a few.

- Wait until the last minute to add a **finishing touch** by tossing with dressing and then adding some seeds, herbs, microgreens, and/or edible flowers to top it off.

- If you're out of ideas, **explore the local farmer's market** or wander through the grocery store and buy one new ingredient to add to your salad every week. Choose a plant you've never tried before or haven't eaten in a while and challenge yourself to make a meal featuring this new "plant of the week." More variety equals more nutrients and gets you closer to that important goal of more than thirty plants per week.

- Grab a fork, give thanks for all this microbe-boosting fresh food, and **dig in!**

———

Cabbage-Kale Crunch
Serves 4

Keep your gut healthy and your microbes humming a happy song with this delicious and easy kale and cabbage slaw.

Ingredients

2 cups shredded kale leaves

2 to 3 tablespoons avocado oil

3 cups finely shredded red cabbage

1 medium carrot, finely shredded

1 medium jalapeño, seeded and minced

½ cup finely chopped fresh cilantro, plus extra for garnish

Juice of 1 lime

1 lime, sliced, for garnish

Sea salt to taste

¼ cup crushed cashews

Method

Massage the kale with 1 tablespoon of the avocado oil. In a large bowl, toss together the kale, cabbage, carrot, jalapeño, and cilantro. Drizzle with the remaining 1 to 2 tablespoons avocado oil and the lime juice. Season with salt to taste and toss again. Top with the crushed cashews and extra cilantro. Serve with sliced lime.

Root Vegetable Salad with Herby Vinaigrette
Serves 4 to 6

This grounding recipe is as flexible as it gets. Use any combination of beets, carrots, parsnips, sweet potatoes, turnips, or rutabaga that you like. Then serve on your preferred mix of leafy greens.

Ingredients
Vegetables

4 cups root vegetables, cubed or sliced in sticks

Olive oil for coating the vegetables

Pinch of salt

¼ cup chopped fresh parsley

8 cups greens (can use a mixture of spinach, spring mix, mâche, arugula)

Dried cranberries and pecans, for toppings

Dressing

¼ cup olive oil

¼ cup balsamic vinegar

1 tablespoon maple syrup

2 teaspoons Dijon mustard

1 to 2 tablespoons chopped fresh herbs (parsley, thyme, and rosemary work well)

Sea salt and freshly ground black pepper to taste

Method
Make the vegetables:

Preheat the oven to 400°F. Line two rimmed baking sheets with parchment paper.

In a large bowl, add the root veggies and mix in the olive oil, pinch of salt, and chopped parsley. Place the vegetables in a single layer on the baking sheets and roast in the oven for 35 to 40 minutes, or until golden brown around the edges and crispy. (The roasting time depends on the thickness of the sliced veggies.) Turn over once halfway through cooking. Remove the vegetables from the oven and cool slightly.

Make the dressing:

While the vegetables are cooling, make the dressing by whisking together the olive oil, vinegar, 1 tablespoon water, the maple syrup, mustard, herbs, salt, and pepper in a small bowl. Place the vegetables on a bed of greens. Add some dried cranberries and pecans and drizzle with the balsamic maple dressing. Store extra dressing in the refrigerator for up to 5 days. Serve warm or at room temperature.

———

Arugula Salad with Quinoa, Avocado, Blueberries, and Walnuts

Serves 4

This salad combines so many good-for-you food groups: leafy greens, healthy plant-based fats, whole grains, fruit, and nuts.

Ingredients
Lemony Vinaigrette

¼ cup freshly squeezed lemon juice

1 tablespoon Dijon mustard

1 teaspoon maple syrup (optional)

1 tablespoon minced shallots

¼ cup olive oil

½ teaspoon sea salt

Freshly ground black pepper

Salad

6 to 8 cups arugula

1 cup blueberries

1 avocado, sliced and cubed

1 cup cooked quinoa

¼ cup chopped walnuts

Method

Make the lemony vinaigrette:

In a small bowl, whisk together the lemon juice, mustard, and maple syrup, if using. Add in the shallots. Slowly combine the olive oil with the dressing mixture and blend until well combined. Season with salt and pepper to taste. Set aside.

Make the salad:

Combine arugula, blueberries, and cubed avocado in a large salad bowl. Next, add the quinoa and mix in to coat all of the ingredients. Pour the dressing over the salad and toss to coat. Top with walnuts. Store any remaining dressing in the refrigerator for up to 5 days.

———

Grilled Peach and White Bean Salad with Basil Vinaigrette

Serves 4

This salad is super versatile: use nectarines, plums, or apricots in place of peaches, which can all be easily tossed onto the grill. Or try mixed leafy greens instead of arugula.

Ingredients

Vinaigrette

¼ cup olive oil

3 tablespoons freshly squeezed lemon juice

1 garlic clove, coarsely chopped

2 teaspoons Dijon mustard

¼ cup fresh basil leaves, packed tightly

2 teaspoons raw honey or maple syrup

½ teaspoon sea salt

Freshly ground black pepper

Salad

2 to 3 ripe peaches, pitted and halved

2 medium zucchinis, sliced lengthwise

Olive oil or avocado oil for grilling

1 cup cooked white beans

2 cups fresh cherry or grape tomatoes, halved

1 cup cooked corn

4 to 5 cups arugula

¼ cup sliced almonds, toasted

Sea salt and freshly ground pepper

Method

Make the vinaigrette:

Add the olive oil, lemon juice, garlic, mustard, basil, honey, salt, and pepper to the bowl of a blender (or place all of the ingredients in a large bowl and use a handheld immersion blender). Blend until smooth and creamy. Adjust the seasonings to taste.

Make the salad:

Preheat the grill to medium-high. Brush the peaches and the zucchini with oil. Arrange the peaches and zucchini on the grates and cook for 3 to 4 minutes, until charred, flipping halfway through. (This is a rough estimate as it depends on the thickness of the slices.) Remove from the grill and set aside.

In a large bowl, mix together the beans, tomatoes, and corn. Toss with 1 to 2 tablespoons of dressing until lightly coated. Add the arugula to the bottom of a tray or large bowl. Layer the bean-tomato-corn mixture next.

Then place the grilled peaches and zucchini on top. Next, sprinkle on the sliced almonds and drizzle with the basil vinaigrette. Season with salt and pepper to taste. Toss all together and serve immediately.

———

Beet, Fennel, and Orange Salad with Cumin Lime Dressing
Serves 4

Beets are high in inulin and help promote the growth of good gut bacteria. The cumin lime dressing gives a zesty touch to the already flavorful combination of ingredients.

Ingredients
1 large bunch of leafy greens of choice (arugula or butter lettuce work well)
2 medium-large beets, roasted and peeled
2 fennel bulbs, trimmed, quartered, and sliced thin
1 large navel orange, peeled and sliced in rounds
¼ cup walnuts
3 tablespoons fresh mint
¼ cup freshly squeezed lime juice
2 teaspoons maple syrup
¼ teaspoon cumin, or to taste
1 tablespoon fresh cilantro, chopped
Sea salt and freshly ground black pepper to taste
¼ cup olive oil

Method
Add the leafy greens to a large bowl. Next, combine the beets, fennel, orange slices, walnuts, and mint and add to the leafy greens. In a small bowl, whisk the lime juice, maple syrup, cumin, cilantro, salt, and pepper. Slowly drizzle in the olive oil and whisk again. Toss the salad with the dressing and serve immediately.

HEARTY ONE-POT DISHES

Moroccan Spiced Chickpeas
Serves 6 to 8

This is a very flexible recipe that's easy to modify. For a heartier version, add a scoop of quinoa or brown rice before serving. Out of zucchini or squash? Just leave it out! Not into spicy? Forget the cayenne! Too much garlic? Two cloves will do! In the mood for a soup instead? Just thin it out with a little broth.

Ingredients

2 tablespoons olive oil

1 onion, chopped

3 garlic cloves, minced

3 stalks celery, sliced

1 teaspoon ground oregano

1 teaspoon ground cumin

1 teaspoon paprika

1 teaspoon ground coriander

Pinch of cayenne

1 tablespoon fresh turmeric, grated, or 1 teaspoon ground

4 carrots, sliced in rounds

1 zucchini, sliced

1 yellow squash, sliced

Freshly ground black pepper to taste

3 cups cooked chickpeas or 2 (15-ounce) BPA-free cans, drained and rinsed

6 cups vegetable stock

1 teaspoon sea salt, or to taste

1 cup fresh herbs (any combination of parsley and cilantro), plus extra for
   garnish

3 cups loosely packed fresh spinach

Juice of 2 lemons

1 lemon, sliced

Method

In a large pot, heat the olive oil over medium heat. Add the onion, garlic, and celery and sauté for about 6 minutes, until tender. Next, mix in the oregano, cumin, paprika, coriander, cayenne, and turmeric and cook for 1 minute. Add the carrots, zucchini, squash, and pepper and sauté for about 5 minutes, until softened.

Next, add the cooked chickpeas and stir the mixture until covered with the spices. Pour in the stock and add the salt and more pepper. Bring to a boil over high heat, then reduce the heat to a simmer and cover. Cook for 30 to 35 minutes, or until the vegetables can be pierced through with a fork.

Turn off the heat and add in the herbs and spinach. Mix with a spoon to distribute evenly. Add the lemon juice and stir again. Adjust the seasonings to taste. Serve hot with lemon slices and fresh herbs on top.

———

Cauliflower Tikka Masala
Serves 4

If there was ever a dish to convince you that plant-based food can be full of flavor and satisfying, too, this is it! The seasoned cauliflower combines with healing spices and a hearty sauce that will leave you feeling comforted and nourished from the inside out. Coconut milk is used in place of dairy for a lighter take on this Indian-inspired meal.

Ingredients

2 teaspoons garam masala

1 teaspoon ground turmeric

1 teaspoon ground cumin

1 teaspoon sweet paprika

1 teaspoon fine sea salt

1 medium head of cauliflower (about 2 pounds), cored and cut into florets

¼ cup olive oil

½ yellow onion, finely chopped

2 garlic cloves, minced

2 teaspoons peeled and finely grated fresh ginger

2 tablespoons tomato paste

1½ cups crushed tomatoes (1 [14.5-ounce] can or jar)

1 cup coconut milk or coconut cream

1 tablespoon freshly squeezed lime juice, or to taste (can substitute lemon
    juice)

¼ cup finely chopped fresh cilantro, plus extra leaves for garnish

Steamed basmati or brown rice, for serving

Method

Preheat the oven to 450°F. In a small bowl, whisk together the garam masala, turmeric, cumin, paprika, and salt. Put the cauliflower on a large, rimmed baking sheet and drizzle with 2 tablespoons of the olive oil. Toss until evenly coated. Add 1 tablespoon of the spice mixture and toss until evenly coated. Spread the cauliflower into an even layer. Roast for about 12 minutes, until the cauliflower is nicely golden and crisp-tender, turning once about halfway through.

Meanwhile, warm the remaining 2 tablespoons of olive oil in a large saucepan over medium heat. Add the onion and cook, stirring occasionally, for about 5 minutes, until tender. Add the garlic and ginger and cook for 1 more minute, then add the tomato paste and remaining spice mixture. Cook, stirring, for about 1 minute, until fragrant.

Add the tomatoes and ¼ cup water and stir to combine, scraping up any browned bits from the pan bottom. Bring to a boil, then reduce the heat to low and simmer, stirring occasionally, for about 8 minutes, until the sauce is fragrant and thickens slightly. Add the roasted cauliflower, coconut milk, and lime juice and simmer until the cauliflower is done to your liking and the sauce is warmed through. Stir in the cilantro.

Serve with rice, garnished with cilantro leaves.

Tips

Want it spicy? Add ½ teaspoon cayenne pepper when you add the spice mixture to the pan with the tomato paste.

Want a smooth sauce? Puree with an immersion blender before adding the cauliflower.

Want more protein? Add in cooked red lentils for a more filling meal.

———

Mexican Spiced Quinoa Vegetable Stew
Serves 6 to 8

Self-care comes in many forms, and sometimes it's in the shape of a big pot of nourishing stew. Whip up a fresh batch at the beginning of the week to have a cozy bowl available any time you need a dose of TLC. Filled with healing spices, plant-based protein, vibrant veggies, and leafy greens, this dish will warm and nourish you inside and out.

Ingredients

2 tablespoons olive oil or avocado oil

1 onion, chopped

2 large carrots, thinly sliced

2 stalks celery, thinly sliced

2 garlic cloves, minced

2 teaspoons cumin

1 teaspoon oregano

1 teaspoon paprika

½ teaspoon crushed red pepper flakes, plus extra for garnish

1½ teaspoons sea salt, or to taste

4 to 5 cups vegetables, chopped (zucchini, yellow squash, red bell pepper, and cauliflower work well)

2 tablespoons tomato paste

6 cups vegetable broth, plus more as needed (see Note)

½ cup cooked quinoa

1½ cups cooked black beans or 1 (15-ounce) BPA-free can, drained and rinsed

1 cup cherry or grape tomatoes, halved

½ cup chopped fresh cilantro, plus extra for garnish

4 cups fresh spinach, loosely packed

Juice of 1 large lime

1 lime, cut into 6 to 8 wedges

1 avocado, sliced

Method

Heat the oil in a Dutch oven or large pot over medium heat. Add the onion, carrots, and celery and sauté for 5 to 6 minutes, until tender. Next, add the garlic, cumin, oregano, paprika, red pepper flakes, and salt. Cook for 1 minute, until the mixture is well coated. Add in the 4 to 5 cups chopped vegetables of choice and sauté for 5 minutes, until softened.

Add the tomato paste, broth, and 1 cup water and bring to a boil (adjust liquid amount if necessary). Reduce to a simmer, cover, and cook for 10 minutes. Add the quinoa and black beans and cook for an additional 15 minutes or until all of the vegetables can be pierced with a fork. Turn off the heat and add in the tomatoes, ¼ cup of the cilantro, and the spinach. Mix with a spoon to distribute evenly. Squeeze the lime juice into the pot and season with additional salt and pepper to taste. Serve hot with an extra squeeze of lime, the remaining ¼ cup cilantro, and crushed red pepper flakes. Garnish each bowl with a wedge of lime, sliced avocado, and extra cilantro.

Note

Use additional broth if the soup becomes too thick after refrigerating.

Lentils and Roasted Carrots with a Lemon-Herb Tahini Sauce

Serves 4 to 6

This dish is delicious served over either leafy greens or whole grains (or both!). If you're short on time, just make the lentils to eat with other meals, or roast a tray of carrots for a gorgeous side dish. The tahini sauce can be used on veggie burgers or roasted vegetables, or as a crudité dip.

Ingredients

Lemon-Herb Tahini Sauce

¼ cup tahini

Juice of ½ lemon

1 teaspoon finely chopped mixed fresh herbs, such as basil, chives, oregano, parsley

½ teaspoon sea salt

Lentils

1½ cups dried green lentils

1 teaspoon fine sea salt, plus more to taste

2 tablespoons olive oil

1 tablespoon freshly squeezed lemon juice, or to taste

Freshly ground black pepper

Roasted Carrots

2 bunches (about 24 ounces) of small carrots

2 tablespoons olive oil

½ teaspoon cumin

Sea salt and freshly ground black pepper

For Serving

4 cups packed leafy greens or cooked whole grains

Fresh cilantro leaves, for garnish

Method

Make the lemon-herb tahini sauce:

In a bowl, whisk together the tahini, lemon juice, 1 tablespoon water, and the herbs. Add additional water as needed to thin the sauce to a smooth, spreadable consistency. Taste and season with salt. Set aside.

Preheat the oven to 425°F.

Make the lentils:

In a saucepan over high heat, bring 6 cups water, the lentils, and the salt to a boil. Reduce the heat to medium-low and simmer for 20 to 30 minutes, stirring occasionally and skimming any scum from the top, until the lentils are tender but retain their shape (the amount of time depends on how fresh the lentils are). Drain in a colander, then return to the pan. Stir in the olive oil, lemon juice, and salt and pepper to taste. Set aside.

Make the roasted carrots:

While the lentils are cooking, roast the vegetables. Trim the carrots. Cut in half lengthwise if medium-sized or quarter if large. On a rimmed baking sheet, toss the carrots with the olive oil, then season with the cumin, salt, and pepper.

Roast for 20 to 25 minutes, tossing occasionally, until the carrots are crisp tender and golden around the edges. (Keep an eye on the veggies and remove them as they finish cooking, allowing the remaining veggies to continue roasting as necessary.) Toss the warm carrots with most of the tahini sauce.

To serve:
Divide the leafy greens or cooked grains among individual plates, or mound onto a platter. Top with the lentils and roasted carrots. Spoon the remainder of the tahini sauce over the top. Garnish with cilantro and enjoy!

––––

Skillet Shakshuka
Serves 4

Shakshuka is a fragrant pepper-and-tomato-based Middle Eastern egg dish. The eggs are baked into the warm sauce, then topped with fresh herbs and green onions. The garlic and anti-inflammatory spices enliven the sauce, which you can make up to two days in advance—just warm it back up before you add the eggs.

Ingredients
2 tablespoons olive oil
¼ small yellow onion, finely chopped
1 red bell pepper, cored, seeded, and chopped
2 garlic cloves, minced
1 teaspoon paprika
½ teaspoon chopped fresh or dried oregano
¼ teaspoon ground cumin
Fine sea salt and freshly ground black pepper
2 cups canned whole tomatoes, with their juices
1 cup fresh baby spinach
4 to 6 large eggs
¼ cup crumbled vegan cheese
1 thinly sliced green onion (scallion) (white and green parts)
¼ cup chopped fresh cilantro or flat-leaf parsley

Method

Preheat the oven to 400°F. In a 10-inch ovenproof skillet over medium heat, heat the olive oil. Add the onion and bell pepper and cook for about 7 minutes, until the vegetables are tender and starting to brown, stirring occasionally.

Stir in the garlic, paprika, oregano, cumin, ½ teaspoon salt, and a few grinds of pepper. Cook for about 30 seconds, just until fragrant. Reduce the heat to medium-low and add the tomatoes with their juices, breaking them up with your hands as you add them. Stir to combine.

Bring the mixture to a simmer, then stir in the spinach. Continue to simmer for about 5 minutes, until the spinach is wilted and the sauce is fragrant. (If the sauce is too thick, add a few tablespoons of water.)

Use the back of a big spoon to create 4 to 6 wells in the tomato mixture. Crack an egg into each well and season with a little salt and pepper. Transfer the pan to the oven and bake for about 12 minutes, until the egg whites are barely cooked and the yolks are still runny. (The eggs will continue to cook while you add the garnishes.)

Sprinkle with the vegan cheese, green onions, and cilantro or Italian parsley. Serve immediately.

Tip

For a vegan version, omit the eggs altogether and add seared cubes of tofu or other plant-based protein instead.

FERMENTS

—

Fermented Veggie Guide
Makes 4 pints

Naturally fermented vegetables are packed with an abundance of beneficial bacteria—plus the fiber to keep your gut microbes well fed and working for you. Fermenting your own vegetables may seem intimidating, but it's actually a pretty simple process. All you need are a handful of ingredients plus a little bit of patience to make your own. Be sure to use distilled, spring, or filtered water and non-iodized salt, or the fermentation process may be impeded. You can ferment almost any hard vegetables, such as beets, radishes, carrots, green beans, cucumbers, cauliflower florets, onions, cabbage, or bell peppers. For this basic but incredibly nourishing fermented veggie recipe, you'll need four sterilized pint jars with lids, vegetables, salt, and water. That's it!

Ingredients

1 pound red beets

2 bunches of small radishes

½ pound small carrots

½ pound green beans

4 cups distilled water

2 tablespoons fine sea salt or other non-iodized salt

Method

Peel the beets, halve them lengthwise, and slice them very thinly (about ¹⁄₁₆ inch thick); alternatively, cut them into matchsticks. Stack the beets in one of the pint jars.

Trim the radishes and cut them in halves or quarters, depending on how large they are, or slice them into ⅛-inch-thick slices. Pack them into one of the pint jars.

Trim the carrots and peel or scrub them well. Halve them lengthwise or cut them into sticks; they should come no farther than about 1 inch below the rim of a pint jar. Pack them into one of the jars.

Trim the green beans so they come no farther than about 1 inch below the rim of a pint jar. Tightly pack them into the jar.

In a large glass measuring pitcher or a bowl, stir together the water and salt until the salt dissolves. Pour the salt water over the vegetables, leaving at least 1 inch of space at the top of the jar. Cover the jars tightly and set aside at room temperature. Once a day, open each jar to release the gases produced during fermentation. If any mold or scum form on top, · skim it off. Taste the fermented vegetables, and when they are done to your liking (usually after 3 to 5 days), transfer them to the refrigerator;

chilling will slow down the fermentation. Stored in the refrigerator, the fermented veggies will last for up to 1 month.

Variations:

You can add aromatics like spices, herbs, garlic, ginger, or chilies to add additional flavor to the fermented vegetables. The ingredient amounts below are for each pint:

Beets with 3 slices fresh ginger and ½ teaspoon orange zest

Radishes with 1 sliced garlic clove

Carrots with 1 bay leaf and 1 teaspoon coriander seeds or 3 slices fresh ginger

———

Easy Coconut Milk Kefir

Serves 2

Kefir is a tangy, milk- or water-based drink fermented by a combination of bacteria and yeast and is a rich source of healthy, diverse microbes. You can buy commercial kefir at the store, but this recipe makes a much tastier and healthier version. The symbiotic combination of bacteria and yeast forms "grains" that resemble small cauliflower florets and may contain up to thirty different kinds of helpful bacteria.

Ingredients

½ cup milk kefir grains

2 cups coconut milk

Method

Place the kefir grains in a wide-mouthed quart canning or mason jar and pour in the coconut milk. Lay a square of paper towel across the top and screw down the lid band without the lid. Let the coconut milk sit at room temperature for 12 to 15 hours (less time for warmer temperatures, more time for cooler temperatures), until the milk is thick as a result of culturing by the bacteria in the grains. Use a strainer and spoon to retrieve the cultured coconut milk curds, adding the grains back to the quart jar to be used to make another batch.

SNACKS

———

Lemony Garlic Hummus
Serves 4

Plant-based protein and healthy fat come together in this easy-to-make, nutrient-dense dip. Chop some veggies and whip up this zesty hummus, then serve it up for a satisfying and healthy snack.

Ingredients

1½ cups chickpeas, drained and rinsed

1 large garlic clove, minced

2 tablespoons freshly squeezed lemon juice

¼ cup tahini

2 tablespoons olive oil, plus a drizzle for garnish

½ teaspoon ground cumin

½ teaspoon grated lemon zest, or to taste

Chopped parsley and paprika, for garnish

Method

Add the chickpeas and garlic to the bowl of a high-speed blender or food processor and let it run for 1 minute.

Add the lemon juice, tahini, olive oil, cumin, lemon zest, and 2 tablespoons water and run for 1 more minute. Drizzle with olive oil and sprinkle with parsley and paprika.

Tip

To make a grab-and-go snack: Add about ¼ cup of hummus to the bottom of a 4-ounce mason jar. Fill several jars with vegetable strips and store covered in the refrigerator for up to 3 days.

High-Fiber Trail Mix

Makes 4 cups

This trail mix is an easy, on-the-go snack that tastes delicious, isn't loaded with sugar, and is high in fiber. Pack up a mason jar and store it in your desk, make individual serving packets to throw in your bag, or bring it along on your next hike.

Ingredients

½ cup sunflower seeds

½ cup pumpkin seeds

1 cup walnuts or almonds

1 cup dried apricots (unsulfured)

½ cup coconut flakes

½ cup unsweetened cherries

Method

Mix the sunflower seeds, pumpkin seeds, walnuts, dried apricots, coconut flakes, and unsweetened cherries together in a bowl and store in an airtight container.

Root Veggie Chips with Tahini Dipping Sauce

Serves 4

There is something so satisfying about replacing a store-bought item with a healthier homemade version, and these baked veggie chips are a great example of that. Top them off with a tahini dipping sauce for extra nutrients and anti-inflammatory ingredients like cumin.

Ingredients

Root Veggie Chips (see Notes)

1 large sweet potato

1 Japanese yam

2 large beets

Olive oil or avocado oil to coat (about 1 tablespoon)

1 teaspoon sea salt, or to taste

Tahini Dipping Sauce

½ cup tahini

½ teaspoon garlic powder

½ teaspoon cumin

½ teaspoon sea salt

¼ cup warm water (adjust to desired thickness)

Sprinkle of paprika and a sprig of fresh parsley, for garnish

Method

Make the root veggie chips:

Preheat the oven to 375°F. Line two large baking sheets with parchment paper.

Peel and slice the sweet potato, yam, and beets into thin rounds. This can be done with a handheld slicer or a mandoline on the ¹⁄₁₆-inch setting. Place the sliced veggies in a large mixing bowl and toss with oil so that each round is lightly coated. (This may need to be done in batches.)

Place the sliced veggies in a single layer on the prepared baking sheets. Bake for about 20 minutes, flipping the rounds over after about 12 minutes (see Notes). Remove from the oven when the chips are golden brown around the edges. Let stand for 5 minutes before eating to allow the chips to crisp up. Sprinkle with additional sea salt and other seasonings, if desired. Repeat the baking process with the remaining veggies. Serve in a shallow bowl alongside the tahini dipping sauce.

Best eaten immediately. Store the remaining chips in an airtight container for up to 2 days.

Make the tahini dipping sauce:

In a small mixing bowl, combine the tahini, garlic powder, cumin, and salt. Whisk until smooth. Slowly add in the warm water and whisk until the desired consistency is reached. Adjust the seasonings to taste. Top with paprika and parsley. Serve alongside the chips. Store the remaining sauce in the refrigerator for up to 5 days.

Notes

Other veggie options for making the chips include parsnips, radishes, Yukon Gold potatoes, carrots, rutabagas, and turnips.

The chips can burn easily, and depending on the thickness, the baking time can vary. Check every few minutes after flipping the vegetables and adjust the cooking time accordingly.

———

Two-Way Sweet Potato Toasts
Makes 8 toasts or 4 servings

Sweet potatoes are nutritional powerhouses containing lots of potassium, beta-carotene that your body converts to vitamin A, magnesium, and both soluble and insoluble fiber. Try them with mashed avocado, sliced radish, hempseeds, and a tahini drizzle, or go for a sweet version using your choice of nut butter and berries.

Ingredients

1 large sweet potato (¾ to 1 pound), scrubbed but not peeled
Avocado oil or olive oil for brushing

Savory Toppings

1 ripe avocado, pitted, peeled, and thinly sliced
Fine sea salt
4 small radishes, very thinly sliced
4 teaspoons hempseeds or toasted sesame seeds
½ teaspoon crushed red pepper flakes
½ cup microgreens
Drizzle of tahini or any tahini dressing

Sweet Toppings

¼ cup nut butter of choice
¼ cup fresh berries
4 teaspoons hempseeds
1 teaspoon ground cinnamon

Method

Preheat the oven to 425°F. Line a baking sheet with parchment paper. Trim the ends from the sweet potato, then cut a very thin slice off lengthwise down one side. Place the sweet potato sliced-edge down; this will help hold it in place when you slice it.

Cut the sweet potato into ¼-inch-thick slabs; you should have 8 slices. Lightly brush the slices on both sides with oil. Arrange in a single layer on the prepared baking sheet so they are not touching. Bake for 20 to 25 minutes, until tender and browned around the edges, turning once or twice during the baking.

Divide the sweet potato slices among 4 individual plates, with 2 slices per serving.

Add the savory toppings:

Top 1 slice of sweet potato toast on each plate with avocado slices, dividing them evenly among the slices. Lightly mash the avocado with a fork, then sprinkle lightly with salt. Top the avocado with radish slices, hempseeds, red pepper flakes, and microgreens, dividing them evenly. Sprinkle with a little more salt and drizzle with tahini or the tahini sauce. Serve.

Add the sweet toppings:

Top the other slice of sweet potato toast on each plate with nut butter, dividing it evenly among the slices. Top the nut butter with berries, hempseeds, and cinnamon, dividing them evenly. Drizzle with a little more nut butter if desired. Serve.

Store any remaining slices in a container in the refrigerator and reheat or toast in a toaster to eat throughout the week.

Tip

You can top the savory toast with an egg or smoked salmon and capers. For another sweet variety, experiment with nut butter, sliced bananas, and cacao nibs. The possibilities are endless!

DESSERTS

Zesty Chia Pudding
Serves 2

Despite being in the dessert section, this healthy treat is made from fibrous chia seeds that help fill you up and feed your microbes.

Ingredients

1 cup plant-based milk (ideally coconut milk)

1 tablespoon maple syrup, or to taste

Finely grated zest of 1 lemon, plus extra for garnish

½ teaspoon vanilla extract

Pinch of fine sea salt

¼ cup chia seeds

Fresh fruit, for serving (optional)

Method

In a small bowl, combine the milk, maple syrup, lemon zest, vanilla, and salt. Whisk to blend. Add the chia seeds and whisk until well combined. Cover the bowl or transfer the mixture to a mason jar, making sure the pudding has room to expand. Refrigerate for at least 3 hours or up to overnight, ideally stirring once about 2 hours after the pudding starts to thicken, to help distribute the chia seeds evenly.

Delicious on its own or serve with fresh fruit and store any remaining pudding in the refrigerator for up to 5 days.

"Cookie Dough" Balls
Makes sixteen 1½-inch balls

Who's got their hands in the cookie jar? You do now, and you can feel good about munching on these incredibly delicious raw "cookie dough" balls. One bite, and you won't even miss the sugar, flour, or processed ingredients. Filled with healthy fats, protein, and other nutrient-dense ingredients, these "cookies" will do the trick as a midday pick-me-up or satisfying dessert.

Ingredients

1 cup cashews

½ cup pecans

½ cup walnuts

¼ cup goji berries

1 tablespoon coconut oil

2 tablespoons maple syrup

½ teaspoon ground cinnamon

1 teaspoon vanilla extract

Pinch of sea salt

2 tablespoons cacao nibs

Method

Place the cashews, pecans, and walnuts in the bowl of a food processor and process until they are in pieces but not a powder. Add in the goji berries, coconut oil, maple syrup, cinnamon, vanilla, and salt. Combine and process until a dough-like consistency begins to form but there are still little chunks of nuts and goji berries remaining. Add in the cacao nibs and pulse a few times to incorporate the nibs.

To make the balls: Use a small scooper (about 1½ inches in diameter) or roll 1 tablespoon at a time in your hands. Because the mixture is mostly nuts, it will feel oily if you roll the balls by hand. Make sure to pack the dough tightly against the scooper or in your hands before placing them on a plate or tray. Put in the freezer for 30 minutes to set. Store in the refrigerator up to 5 days or in the freezer for up to 2 months (if they last that long!).

Chocolate Orange Mousse
Serves 2 to 3

This combination of chocolate and avocado spiced with a splash of orange and a sprinkling of cinnamon whips up into the creamiest, dreamiest dessert that feels just as good as it tastes!

Ingredients

2 ripe avocados, peeled and pitted

¼ cup raw cacao powder

1 to 2 tablespoons coconut milk (adjust to desired consistency)

4 to 5 tablespoons maple syrup

½ teaspoon vanilla extract

Juice from ½ orange (about 1 tablespoon)

1 teaspoon orange zest, plus more for topping

½ teaspoon ground cinnamon

Pinch of sea salt (do not skip this!)

Method

Place the avocados, cacao powder, coconut milk, maple syrup, vanilla, orange juice, 1 teaspoon orange zest, cinnamon, and salt in the bowl of a food processor or high-speed blender. Slowly add in a splash or two of coconut milk until the mixture reaches the desired consistency, scraping down the sides as necessary (this is a thick dessert).

Place the mousse in the refrigerator for at least 30 minutes to let the flavors set before serving. Store in the refrigerator for up to 2 days. Serve in individual small bowls and sprinkle with orange zest.

Skillet Peach Crisp
Serves 6 to 8

A crunchy oat topping, crispy quinoa, and a luscious peach filling come together to create a high-fiber summer party in a skillet!

Ingredients

1 tablespoon melted coconut oil

Oat Topping

1½ cups old-fashioned rolled oats

¼ cup cooked quinoa

¼ cup oat flour

½ cup chopped nuts (almonds, pecans, or hazelnuts work) (optional)

½ teaspoon sea salt

1 tablespoon coconut sugar or maple syrup (coconut sugar makes it a little crispy on top)

¼ cup coconut oil, softened but not melted, plus more for the pan

1 teaspoon vanilla extract

Peach Filling

2 to 3 pounds ripe but semi-firm fresh peaches, peeled, pitted, and cut into ½-inch-thick wedges

1 tablespoon maple syrup, or to taste

1 tablespoon tapioca starch

1 tablespoon freshly squeezed lemon juice

Method

Preheat the oven to 375°F. Grease a 10-inch cast-iron skillet lightly with melted coconut oil.

Make the oat topping:

In a medium bowl, stir together the oats, quinoa, oat flour, nuts (if adding), and salt. Add the coconut sugar, softened coconut oil, and vanilla and stir until the mixture is evenly moistened and clumped. Set aside.

Make the peach filling:

In a medium bowl, toss together the peaches, maple syrup, tapioca starch, and lemon juice. Pour the filling into the prepared cast-iron pan and spread in an even layer. Top with the oat topping. Bake for about 45 minutes, until the peaches are tender, the juices are bubbling, and the topping is crisp and golden brown. Let cool on a wire rack for at least 15 minutes or until it reaches room temperature.

Acknowledgments

Within a few months of the start of the pandemic, clinical studies looking at the health of the gut microbiome as a predictor of outcome from COVID began appearing in the scientific literature, and so did compelling data about the link between stomach acid and the likelihood of infection. This book started with a suggestion from my thoughtful literary agent, Howard Yoon, that an editorial shedding light on some of these gastrointestinal issues might be a useful public service endeavor. With each important scientific article connecting the health of the gut with SARS-CoV-2 outcome, my fascination (obsession, really) with spreading the word among patients, friends, and family grew. Ultimately, it grew into this book, which wouldn't have been possible without my team at Avery, helmed by the amazing Lucia Watson. Lucia's confidence that my hastily crafted proposal written over the weekend at my kitchen table could eventually become a book that would not just educate, but maybe save lives, kept me motivated through the slog of wading through hundreds of research articles and keeping up with a science that was literally changing daily. Douglas Varner, assistant dean for information management at Georgetown University, was the steadfast supplier of much of that information, providing me with monthly summaries of the latest scientific literature on all things COVID and saving me countless hours in time I would have had to spend doing the searches myself. Kathryn Huck came to my rescue at just the right moment with spot-on editorial advice. She helped me wrestle an unwieldy and disorganized first draft into something much more digestible, and did it in the kindest, gentlest way. Leslie Ann Berg, my chief of operations for all the things I do in my professional life when I'm not writing books, was patient and understanding as I missed deadlines and pushed more work her way on other projects, so I'd have more time to spend on this one. Dr. Ida Bergstrom, Mona Sutphen, and Alicia Sokol are more than good friends and helpful readers of chapters—they are my sisters from other misters who cheered me on to the finish line with this book as they have countless other times. Thank you to my husband, Eric, who more than a decade ago encouraged me to "do what you love—run in the woods and write books." And to my beloved Sydney, thanks for never complaining about all the family movie nights I missed while working on this book—we have a lot of catching up to do!

Index

Note: Italicized page numbers indicate material in tables.

Also by
Robynne Chutkan, MD

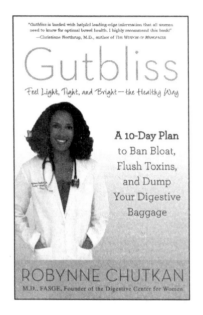

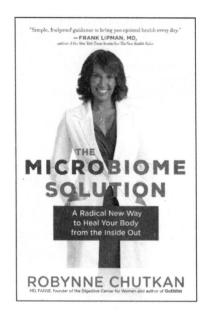

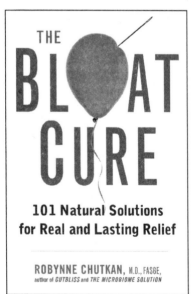